CARDIOLOGY
CLINICAL
QUESTIONS

Notice

Medicine is an ever-changing science. As new research and clinical experience broaden our knowledge, changes in treatment and drug therapy are required. The authors and the publisher of this work have checked with sources believed to be reliable in their efforts to provide information that is complete and generally in accord with the standards accepted at the time of publication. However, in view of the possibility of human error or changes in medical sciences, neither the authors nor the publisher nor any other party who has been involved in the preparation or publication of this work warrants that the information contained herein is in every respect accurate or complete, and they disclaim all responsibility for any errors or omissions or for the results obtained from use of the information contained in this work. Readers are encouraged to confirm the information contained herein with other sources. For example and in particular, readers are advised to check the product information sheet included in the package of each drug they plan to administer to be certain that the information contained in this work is accurate and that changes have not been made in the recommended dose or in the contraindications for administration. This recommendation is of particular importance in connection with new or infrequently used drugs.

CARDIOLOGY CLINICAL QUESTIONS

John P. Higgins, MD, MBA, MPHIL, FACC, FACP, FAHA, FASNC, FSGC
ACSM Certified Clinical Exercise Specialist & Certified Personal Trainer
Associate Professor of Medicine
The University of Texas Health Science Center at Houston (UTHealth)
Director of Exercise Physiology
Memorial Hermann Sports Medicine Institute
Chief of Cardiology, Lyndon B. Johnson General Hospital
Principal Investigator HEARTS
(Houston Early Age Risk Testing & Screening Study)
Houston, Texas

Asif Ali, MD
Clinical Assistant Professor
Division of Cardiovascular Medicine
The University of Texas Health Science Center at Houston (UTHealth)
Memorial Hermann Heart and Vascular Institute
Sub-Clinical Investigator HEARTS
(Houston Early Age Risk Testing & Screening Study)
Houston, Texas

David M. Filsoof, MD
Division of Cardiovasuclar Medicine
Sub-Clinical Investigator of HEARTS
(Houston Early Age Risk Testing & Screening Study)
University of Texas-Houston Health Science Center
Houston, Texas
Mayo School of Graduate Medical Education
Jacksonville, Florida

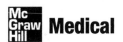

New York   Chicago   San Francisco   Lisbon   London   Madrid   Mexico City
Milan   New Delhi   San Juan   Seoul   Singapore   Sydney   Toronto

The **McGraw·Hill** Companies

Cardiology Clinical Questions

Copyright © 2012 by The McGraw-Hill Companies, Inc. All rights reserved. Printed in the United States of America. Except as permitted under the United States Copyright Act of 1976, no part of this publication may be reproduced or distributed in any form or by any means, or stored in a data base or retrieval system, without the prior written permission of the publisher.

3 4 5 6 7 8 9 0   DOC/DOC   16 15 14 13 12

ISBN 978-0-07-174898-8
MHID 0-07-174898-9

This book was set in Plantin by Thomson Digital.
The editors were James Shanahan and Brian Kearns.
The production supervisor was Catherine Saggese.
Project management was provided by Aakriti Kathuria, Thomson Digital.
The designer was Eve Siegel; the cover designer was Anthony Landi.
Cover image: Fluorescent light micrograph of beating heart cells.
Credit: Roger J. Bick and Brian J. Poindexter/UT-Houston
    Medical School/Photo Researchers, Inc.
RR Donnelley was printer and binder.

This book is printed on acid-free paper.

Library of Congress Cataloging-in-Publication Data
Higgins, John P.
  Clinical questions : cardiology / John P. Higgins, Asif Ali, David M. Filsoof.
    p. ; cm.
  Cardiology
  Includes bibliographical references.
  ISBN-13: 978-0-07-174898-8 (soft cover : alk. paper)
  ISBN-10: 0-07-174898-9 (soft cover : alk. paper)
  I. Ali, Asif, 1974- II. Filsoof, David M. III. Title. IV. Title:
Cardiology.
  [DNLM: 1. Heart Diseases—diagnosis—Examination Questions. 2. Heart
Diseases—therapy—Examination Questions. 3. Diagnostic Techniques,
Cardiovascular—Examination Questions. WG 18.2]
  LC classification not assigned
  616.1'20076—dc23
                                                    2011034477

McGraw-Hill books are available at special quantity discounts to use as premiums and sales promotions, or for use in corporate training programs. To contact a representative please e-mail us at bulksales@mcgraw-hill.com.

CONTENTS

Section IV. Cardiac Diseases

Section V. Examination

Section VI. Arrhythmias

Section VII. Congenital Heart Diseases

Section VIII. Heart Failure and Hypertension

FACULTY ADVISORS

Faiyaz Ahmed, MD
Resident Physician, Department of Family Mecicine
The Toledo Hospital
Family Medicine
Toledo, Ohio

Sajid A. Ali, MD
Department of Internal Medicine
St. John Hospital and Medical Center
Grosse Pointe, Michigan

Mohammad Ghalichi, MD
Senior Advisory Editor
Department of Internal Medicine - Cardiology
University of Texas at Houston
Houston, Texas

Brian E. Gulbis, PharmD
Cardiovascular Clinical Pharmacist
Memorial Hermann Texas Medical Center
Houston, Texas

PREFACE

After years of cardiology consultations, Dr. John P. Higgins realized that many of the same questions were constantly raised, yet the answers were changing as new medical research accrued. He also noted that many students, residents, fellows, and attending physicians had difficulties translating the up-to-date knowledge into practical diagnostic solutions. The truly useful data, while not inaccessible, was tucked away deep in many papers and research reports. In addition, many of the guidelines, books, or software available to assist diagnosis were topic-driven rather than the Frequently Asked Questions (FAQ) format as followed in this text. The vision for the book was to change the approach to diagnosis problem solving by using a simple tool that organized, synthesized, and hence provided a comprehensive epiphany in the form of a point-of-care tool.

Dr. Asif Ali collaborated to bring his expertise in medical animation education and information technology to help develop the format and layout of the book. Dr. David M. Filsoof added to the questions along with chapter revisions and development.

The team holds firmly to the belief that the application of comprehensively collated information is the pivot on which all good diagnostic decisions are made. The process to accomplish this followed the following flow path:

Question ⟶ Data ⟶ Synthesis ⟶ Solution

The platforms for the practical application of this work will be book, computer, and handheld pocket digital assistant formats. Nine areas have been collated for this text, namely:

- Diagnostic Testing
- Acute Coronary Syndrome
- Valvular Disease
- Cardiac Diseases
- Examination
- Arrhythmias
- Congenital Heart Diseases
- Heart failure and Hypertension
- Medications

This book and its chapter selection evolved as a major collection of clinical questions in cardiology (along with their answers), based on the frequency of consult questions the authors were asked over the past few years in Boston (veterans administration and private teaching hospital) and three Texas hospitals (private teaching hospital, county hospital, and a specialist cancer hospital).

While the book outlines several cases where specialized referral and corrective surgery is required, it has a strong bias toward using non-invasive gold standard diagnostic strategies and available medications. The goal is to empower the doctor to get his or her patient to the best solution as efficiently and effectively as possible. The authors seek to take a plethora of information, form it into something useful, and pare down information overload.

In 1995 Harvard Business School Professor Clayton M. Christensen and Joseph Bower coined the term *disruptive technologies*. In 2003 Christensen revised this term to *disruptive innovation*. We believe this book takes on the spirit of a disruptive innovation for it projects a business model that seeks to provide a new improved service, in a way the market does not expect, for a new larger customer audience, and it threatens the status quo with its disruptive impacts. Our model seeks to simulate the consultation process and proceeds directly from an alchemy of questions toward the critical data that must be obtained, and outlines the procedure to reach solutions to the questions.

Relative to each chapter the "Key Concept" section describes and defines the major decision factors impacting the goal of the consult question. This sets the stage to gather pertinent information. The "History" and "Physical Exam" sections focus on important historical data and the signs to look for pertaining to the consult question. The "ECG," "Imaging," and "Lab" sections aim to focus on findings that help narrow the differential based on results and diagnostic tests performed to make the diagnosis. The "Synthesis" section organizes the information into the core components that will be required for the equations that follow. The "Epiphany" section provides the equation into which the synthesized facts are inserted and the resulting solution is clearly stated in a manner that allows point-of-care management. The "Pearls" section provides factual information that is related to the consult question assisting consultants in educating personnel on key teaching take-home points. The "Discussion" section goes over some key items related to the equations that are often asked. The "Contraindications" section alerts the consultant toward signs to watch for when making their recommendations. The "Evidence & References" section offer evidence-based medicine resources pertaining to the consult question. The objective of this organization of sections is to provide a step-by-step effective approach to answering the consult question. It provides clear and present solutions by incorporating up-to-date evidence-based medicine that adheres to the most current guidelines and consensus statements. In addition, by informing the physicians of the precise pieces of information required to answer the question, it helps them save time by obtaining just those key information, and then plug them into the equations ("Epiphany" section) resulting in a speedy answer. The analogy we use is that imagine there are 100 pearls on a beach regarding the topic the consult question addresses. Rather than pick up all 100, we point out what 10 crucial pearls you need, and help you retrieve them. Then, we tell you how to string these 10 pearls together into a "pearl necklace" —the solution to your question. You save time by using only those critical data in the decision process, and also avoid being inundated with less relevant information,

We believe that this book will enable students, interns, residents, fellows, mid-level providers, physician extenders, and attending physicians to better find correct diagnostic solutions to common cardiology questions that arise, especially while they are rotating on inpatient medical services. We sincerely hope it will lead to faster and quality patient care.

Dr. John P. Higgins
Dr. Asif Ali
Dr. David M. Filsoof
28 June 2011

ACKNOWLEDGMENTS

From Dr. John P. Higgins: To borrow from Shakespeare, I would like to thank all of the actors on my stage: students and colleagues who have inspired me; my brothers and sisters (Michael, Kathy, and Paul) who have encouraged me; my parents (Daniel and Patricia) who have instilled in me the joy of learning; and my soul mate, Catherine, who loves and inspires me every day. All of these actors upon my stage have played their part in this project, and I am thankful to all of you for your contributions. Love you guys ... John

From Dr. Asif Ali: To quote Rumi: Everything in the universe is a pitcher brimming with wisdom and beauty. I want to thank my wife Nishath and kids Nylah, Nadia, and Aneesa for their understanding and support in the writing of this book, my grandmother Ayesha Begum who shaped my foundation in education, and my mother and father who developed my core values and gave me a global perspective in life and medicine.

From Dr. David M. Filsoof: I would like to acknowledge my parents Fred and Mahnaz and brother Nader who have stood by my side and have been a continued source of inspiration, love, and admiration.

I would like to also thank Dr. Catalin Loghin for his time and effort in teaching me all aspects of cardiology, who has continued to be a role model of compassion and empathy toward his patients and profession.

DIAGNOSTIC TESTING

Does my patient need an electrophysiological study?

KEY CONCEPT	The decision to refer a patient for an electrophysiological study is based upon the type of conduction abnormality present.
HISTORY	HPI: Episode of sudden cardiac arrest, palpitations, dyspnea, syncope, fatigue, lightheadedness. PMH: Cardiac arrest, atrioventricular block, atrial fibrillation, atrial flutter, ventricular tachycardia.
ELECTRO-CARDIOGRAM	P waves absent, biphasic "sawtooth" flutter waves present, narrow QRS complex, prolonged PR interval of fixed duration followed by a P wave that fails to conduct to the ventricles, dissociation between P wave and QRS.
SYNTHESIS	**EP** = Refer patient for **E**lectro**P**hysiological study. **RS** = Patient with **R**ecurrent **S**yncope that remains unexplained after an appropriate evaluation. **SND** = Patient with **S**inus **N**ode **D**ysfunction. **S-AVB** = **S**ymptomatic (palpitations, dyspnea, syncope, lightheadedness) patients in whom **A**trio**V**entricular **B**lock is suspected. **IVCD** = **I**ntra**V**entricular **C**onduction **D**elay in symptomatic (palpitations, dyspnea, syncope, lightheadedness) patients. **NCT** = **N**arrow **C**omplex **T**achycardia. **WCT** = **W**ide **C**omplex **T**achycardia. **SRCA** = **S**u**R**vivor of **C**ardiac **A**rrest without obvious reversible cause. **C-ABL** = Patients with symptomatic supraventricular tachycardia due to AVNRT, symptomatic atrial tachyarrhythmias, or ventricular tachycardia amenable to **C**atheter **ABL**ation.
E EPIPHANY	**RS = EP** **SND = EP** **S-AVB = EP** **IVCD = EP** **NCT = EP** **WCT = EP** **SRCA = EP** **C-ABL = EP**

 DISCUSSION	Electrophysiological studies provide valuable diagnostic information as they can determine the mechanisms of arrhythmia and help in the decision of whether drug, device, or ablation therapy is suitable.
 PEARLS	– The most common arrhythmia found by EPS studies is ventricular tachycardia, and the most powerful predictor is an ejection fraction of < 40%.
 REFERENCE	1) Tracy CM, et al. American College of Cardiology/American Heart Association Clinical Competence Statement on Invasive Electrophysiology Studies, Catheter Ablation, and Cardioversion. *Circulation.* 2000;102:2309.

4 DIAGNOSTIC TESTING

When do I need to order a stress test?

KEY CONCEPT	Stress testing is used in diagnosis and prognosis of coronary artery disease. It is done via exercise (treadmill, bicycle) or pharmacologic agents (adenosine, persantine, dobutamine).
HISTORY	Patients with symptoms of known/probable ischemic heart disease, stable angina controlled by medicine. The most important clinical finding is chest pain.
PHYSICAL EXAM	Determine if the patient has functional capacity to perform exercise or will need pharmacologic aid to achieve stress.
ELECTRO-CARDIOGRAM	J point depression of 0.1 mV or more and/or ST segment slope of 1 mV/s in 3 consecutive beats (during stress).
IMAGING	Echocardiogram-check LVEF, wall motion abnormalities, hypertrophy.
SYNTHESIS	**CAD** = **C**oronary **A**rtery **D**isease. Patients with intermediate pretest probability of CAD based on age, sex, and symptoms. **RA** = **R**isk **A**ssessment and prognosis of symptomatic patients of those with CAD. Initial evaluation for CAD, changes in clinical status, unstable angina free of symptoms. **POST-MI** = Testing after **M**yocardial **I**nfarction. Prognostic assessment before discharge/evaluation of medical therapy, activity prescription, and rehabilitation. **CARDIO** = **CARDIO**pulmonary exercise testing. Evaluation of exercise capacity and response to therapy and to differentiate in cardiac vs. pulmonary limitations of capacity. **REVASC** = Before and after **REVASC**ularization. Demonstrate proof of ischemia before revascularization and evaluation of recurrent symptoms to suggest ischemia after revascularization. **ST** = Refer patient for **S**tress **T**est.
E EPIPHANY	**CAD = ST** **RA = ST** **POST-MI = ST** **CARDIO = ST** **REVASC = ST**

 DISCUSSION	Stress testing is used to assess the probability and extent of coronary disease by evoking inducible ischemia and ultimately aids in therapy strategies. Sensitivity is 60–70%, and specificity is 60–80%. Patients with possible CAD and symptoms of ischemia should have stress testing to assess the probability of a cardiac event. There are no indications for routine testing in asymptomatic patients without CAD or risk factors, valvular heart disease. Patients at extremely low risk for coronary artery disease should not be referred for stress testing. Due to the very low pre-test probability, a false-positive is more likely than a true-positive, which will then prompt further (often invasive) testing and subject the patient to potential unessessary harm.
 PEARLS	*Contraindications:* Absolute—Active myocardial infarction, unstable angina, uncontrolled arrhythmias, severe symptomatic aortic stenosis, aortic dissection, decompensated heart failure, pulmonary embolism, myopericarditis. Relative—Left main disease, stenotic valvular diseases, electrolyte imbalances, HTN > 200 mm Hg, HOCM, AV blocks,
 REFERENCE	1) Fraker TD Jr, et al. 2007 chronic angina focused update of the ACC/AHA 2002 Guidelines for the management of patients with chronic stable angina. *Circulation.* 2007;116:2762. 2) Lee TH, et al. Noninvasive tests in patients with stable coronary artery disease. *N Engl J Med.* 2001;344:1840.

What are the indications/criteria for myocardial perfusion imaging?

 KEY CONCEPT	Myocardial perfusion imaging provides three-dimensional information by injecting radioisotopes in the patient that binds to specific tissues (myocardium) to deliver information about myocardial perfusion, thickness, contractility, stroke volume, ejection fraction, and cardiac output during parts of the cardiac cycle.
 HISTORY	Patient presents with chest pain, arrhythmias, and acute coronary syndrome, or for evaluation and risk stratification. PM Hx/PSx Hx: Hypertension, aortic dissection, kidney failure, cirrhosis, congenital heart diseases, HOCM, previous MI, history of CAD.
 SYNTHESIS	**MPI** = Refer patient for **M**yocardial **P**erfusion **I**maging. **EVAL** = **EVAL**uation of chest pain/acute chest pain/new heart failure: Intermediate/high pretest for CAD in patients unable to exercise or uninterpretable ECG for patients with no ST elevation and negative cardiac enzymes. **DETECT** = **DETECT**ion of CAD: moderate CHD risk (Framingham), patients with no prior CAD evaluation and no planned cardiac catheterization. **RISK-ASS** = **RISK ASS**essment: for airline pilots, high CHD risk (Framingham), known CAD on cardiac catheterization or prior SPECT in patients who have not been revascularized or patients with worsening symptoms, or >2 years from last study to evaluate for worsening disease, Agatston score >400, stenosis of unclear significance, intermediate Duke treadmill score, intermediate perioperative risk predictor or poor exercise tolerance (<4 METS) for high and intermediate risk surgery, thrombolytic therapy administered but not planning to undergo catheterization in patients with hemodynamically stable STEMI or patients with NSTEMI not planning to undergo early catheterization, evaluation of chest pain post-revascularzation, >5 years post-revascularization. **ISCH-VIAB** = Assessment of **VIAB**ility/**ISCH**emia: known CAD on catheterization, patient eligibly for catheterization. **LVFUNC** = Assessment of **V**entricular **FUNC**tion: nondiagnostic echo, baseline and serial measurements when using cardiotoxic therapies (doxorubicin).
 EPIPHANY	**EVAL = MPI** **DETECT = MPI** **RISK-ASS = MPI** **ISCH-VIAB = MPI** **LVFUNC = MPI**

 DISCUSSION	An appropriate indication does not mean that this is the first choice of testing for a particular patient. There will be indications to perform procedures based on patient-specific and condition-specific data not on this list. The major indications include diagnosis of CAD, identification and degree of coronary artery disease in patients with a positive history, risk stratification in patients who are at risk of having ACS/MI, and for post-intervention evaluation of the heart.
 PEARLS	Sensitivity is 85%, and specificity is 72% for detecting ischemia. If an area of myocardium shows an unchanged diminished tracer even after injection at rest, the defect most likely represents scar or viable, underperfused myocardium. Medications such as calcium channel–blocking drugs and beta-blocking drugs that may alter the heart rate and blood pressure response to exercise should be withheld if possible prior to the MPI test. Negative consequences include risk of procedure from radiation or contrast exposure and poor test performance. Contraindications to testing are unstable angina, acute myocardial infarction (MI) within 2–4 days of testing, uncontrolled systemic hypertension, untreated life-threatening arrhythmias, uncompensated congestive heart failure, advanced atrioventricular block acute myocarditis, acute pericarditis, severe mitral or aortic stenosis, severe obstructive cardiomyopathy, and acute systemic illness.
 REFERENCE	1) ACCF/ASNC Appropriateness Criteria for Single-Photon Emission Computed Tomography Myocardial Perfusion Imaging. *J Am Coll Cardiol.* 2005;46:1587–1605. 2) Ritchie J, Bateman TM, Bonow RO, et al. Guidelines for clinical use of cardiac radionuclide imaging. A report of the AHA/ACC Task Force on Assessment of Diagnostic and Therapeutic Cardiovascular Procedures. Committee on Radionuclide Imaging, developed in collaboration with the American Society of Nuclear Cardiology. *Circulation.* 1995;91:1278–1303. 3) Schlant RC, Friesinger GC, Leonard JJ. Clinical competence in exercise testing. A statement for physicians from the ACP/ACC/AHA Task Force on Clinical Privileges in Cardiology. *J Am Coll Cardiol.* 1990;16:1061–1065. 4) Updated imaging guidelines for nuclear cardiology procedures, part 1. *J Nucl Cardiol.* 2001;8(1):G5–G58.

Should I refer my patient for coronary angiography?

KEY CONCEPT	The decision to refer a patient for coronary angiography is based on the degree and symptoms of myocardial ischemia.
HISTORY	HPI: Patient with chest pain or evidence of myocardial ischemia. PMH: Coronary artery disease (CAD), congestive heart failure (CHF), myocardial infarction (MI), congenital heart disease (CHD), angina. PSH: Percutaneous coronary intervention (PCI), valve repair.
ELECTRO-CARDIOGRAM	ST-elevation, ST-depression, deep Q waves (>1 mm), poor R wave progression, left bundle branch block (LBBB).
IMAGING	ECHO: Left ventricular ejection fraction (LVEF) <35%, wall motion abnormality, left ventricular dilatation.
SYNTHESIS	**CA** = Refer for **C**oronary **A**ngiography with possible intervention. **SAML** = **S**table **A**ngina but with **M**arked **L**imitation of physical activity, ie, cannot walk 2 blocks or 1 flight of stairs without chest discomfort. **UA** = **U**nstable **A**ngina refractory to medical therapy or with recurrent symptoms after initial stabilization, chest pain > 20 minutes, ST changes (>=1 mm), pathological q waves, pulmonary edema, or age > 65. **RVS** = Acute stent closure within 24 hours of PCR and/or recurrent angina or HR within 9 months of PCR. **AMI1** = Patient within 12 hours of onset of symptoms of ST elevation MI or beyond 12 hours if ischemic symptoms persist, where CA can be performed in a timely fashion (door to catheterization time < 90 minutes). **AMI2** = Patients < 75 years within 36 hours of a STEMI, who develops cardiogenic shock and can be revascularized within 18 hours of the onset of shock. **AMI3** = Persistent episodes of symptomatic ischemia with or without ECG changes; myocardial ischemia provoked by minimal exertion during recovery from MI; or ischemia at low levels of exercise with ECG changes (STD >= 1 mm) or imaging abnormalities. **AMI** = **AMI**1, **AMI**2, or **AMI**3. **CHFI** = **CHF** due to systolic dysfunction with angina, regional wall motion abnormalities, or evidence of myocardial ischemia when revascularization is being considered. **VLV** = Prior to valve repair in patients with chest discomfort, ischemia by noninvasive imaging, multiple risk factors for CAD, or infective endocarditis with coronary embolism. **CHDI** = Prior to correction of **CHD** in patients with chest discomfort or evidence of CAD; unexplained cardiac arrest in young patients; or prior to correction of coronary anomaly (congenital coronary stenosis, arteriovenous fistula).

E EPIPHANY	**SAML = CA** **UA = CA** **RVS = CA** **AMI = CA** **VLV = CA** **CHFI = CA** **CHDI = CA**
DISCUSSION	Coronary angiography is used to define the degree of coronary artery patency and the extent of coronary artery disease. Patients at risk for an adverse cardiac event should undergo coronary angiography to determine the appropriate mode of therapy.
CONTRA-INDICATIONS	– Patients at risk for renal failure from contrast should be hydrated with IV .45 saline at 75 cc/hour prior to undergoing coronary angiography.
PEARLS	– The risk of death, myocardial infarction, or other major embolization during coronary angiography is < 2%.
REFERENCE	1) Scanlon P, et al. ACC/AHA guidelines for coronary angiography. *J Am Coll Cardiol.* 1999;33:1756–1824.

When should I order an echocardiogram on my patient, and which type should I order?

KEY CONCEPT	Echocardiogram is an imaging modality used to evaluate cardiac structure, function, and pathology.
HISTORY	HPI: Patient with chest pain, arrhythmia, murmur, dyspnea, or baseline cardiac function evaluation. PMH: Hypertension (HTN), coronary artery disease (CAD), myocardial infarction (MI), congestive heart failure (CHF), valvular disease, congenital heart disease (CHD), cardiomyopathy. SH: Alcohol, smoking. FH: Marfans disease, hypertrophic cardiomyopathy (HCM).
PHYSICAL EXAM	New murmur, elevated jugular venous pressure, prominent right ventricular impulse, abdominal bruit.
SYNTHESIS	**TTE** = Trans**T**horacic **E**chocardiogram. **TEE** = Trans**E**sophageal **E**chocardiogram. **STE** = **ST**ress **E**chocardiogram. **GSAF** = **G**eneral **S**tructure **A**nd **F**unction = symptoms due to cardiac etiology, suspected coronary artery disease, suspected congenital heart disease, sustained or nonsustained supraventricular or ventricular tachycardia, LV function following MI, pulmonary HTN. **ACUTE** = **ACUTE** setting = hemodynamic instability, evaluation of chest pain with nondiagnostic ECG or labs, respiratory failure with suspected cardiac etiology, complications from MI, known/suspected pulmonary embolus to guide therapy. **VALV** = **VALV**ular function = evaluation of a murmur with suspicion of valvular disease, yearly follow-up of valvular disease, valvular disease with change in clinical status, prosthetic valves, infective endocarditis. **AORT** = **AORT**ic disease = Marfans disease, evaluation of proximal aortic root. **HD** = **H**eart **D**isease = evaluation of hypertensive heart disease, initial and routine evaluation of CHF and HCM, evaluation of suspected cardiomyopathy, screening for inherited cardiomyopathy, baseline and serial evaluation for therapy with cardiotoxic agents. **IE** = Suspected **I**nfective **E**ndocarditis or its complication, persistent fever with intracardiac device with suspicion of infective endocarditis. **GUIDE** = To **GUIDE** during cardiac intervention. **CVERS** = Prior to Cardio**VERS**ion in atrial fibrillation/flutter and/or follow-up after anticoagulation. **REPAIR** = Suitability of valve **REPAIR**. **AC-AORT** = Further investigation of **AC**ute **AORT**ic pathology. **PHTN** = **P**ulmonary **H**yper**T**ensio**N**. **DYSP** = **DYSP**nea suspected due to cardiac etiology. **RISK** = **RISK** stratification in coronary artery disease.

 EPIPHANY	**GSAF/ACUTE/VALV/AORT/HD = TTE** **IE/GUIDE/CVERS/REPAIR/AC-AORT = TEE** **PHTN/DYSP/RISK = STE**
 DISCUSSION	While the range of indications for echocardiogram is large, in uncertain indications the individual physician must use clinical judgment to determine the usefulness of echocardiogram for the particular clinical scenario.
 PEARLS	TEE provides enhanced views of atria, mitral valve, great vessels, and prosthetic valves. TEE has shown to have higher sensitivity for detection of endocarditis compared to TTE.
 REFERENCE	1) Douglas PS, et al. ACCF/ASE/ASNC/SCAI/SCCT/SCMR 2007 Appropriateness Criteria for Transthoracic and Transesophageal Echocardiography. *J Am Coll Cardiol.* 2007;50:187.

Does my patient need cardiac pacing?

KEY CONCEPT	The decision to pace a patient is dependent on the presence of symptoms and the type of conduction abnormality.
HISTORY	HPI: Patient with syncope, palpitations, fatigue, dyspnea, decreased exercise tolerance. PMH: Coronary artery disease, myocardial infarction (MI), sinus node disease, arrhythmias. FH: Congenital heart disease, congenital long QT. SH: Alcohol, smoking.
PHYSICAL EXAM	Bradycardia, hypotension.
ELECTRO-CARDIOGRAM	Heart block, bundle branch block, supraventricular tachycardia, prolonged RR interval.
SYNTHESIS	**SYMP** = **SYMP**tomatic patient – syncope, fatigue, lightheadedness, decreased exercise intolerance, palpitations. **ASYM** = **ASYM**ptomatic = no symptoms. **BC** = **B**rady**C**ardia (heart rate < 60 bpm). **PACE** = Refer patient for permanent **PACE**maker placement. **NOT-PACE** = Do **NOT** refer for **PACE**maker. **SND** = **S**inus **N**ode **D**ysfunction. **ABBB** = **A**lternating **B**undle **B**ranch **B**lock. **CSH** = **C**arotid **S**inus **H**ypersensitivity. **NCS** = **N**euro**C**ardiogenic **S**yncope. **PAVB** = **P**ersistent second or third degree **AV B**lock. **RSVT** = **R**ecurrent **S**upra**V**entricular **T**achycardia that fails with drugs or ablation. **RBBB** = **R**ight **B**undle **B**ranch **B**lock. **PRR** = **P**rolonged **RR** intervals. **2DMB** = **2**nd **D**egree **M**obitz type 1 **B**lock. **LAD** = **L**eft **A**xis **D**eviation. **RAVB** = **R**eversible **AV B**locks (sleep apnea, Lyme disease, vagal tone, drugs).

E EPIPHANY	**SND + SYMP + BC = PACE** **SYMP + PAVB = PACE** **ABBB = PACE** **CSH + BC = PACE** **NCS + BC = PACE** **RSVT = PACE** **ASYM + SND = NOT-PACE** **ASYM + BC = NOT-PACE** **ASYM + 2DMB = NOT-PACE** **ASYM + PRR = NOT-PACE** **ASYM + RBBB + LAD = NOT-PACE** **RAVB = NOT-PACE**
DISCUSSION	Several factors must be taken into consideration when selecting the mode of pacing: overall physical condition, exercise capacity, response to exercise, and associated medical problems.
PEARLS	Exclude reversible causes of AV block before considering pacing.
REFERENCE	1) Epstein AE, et al. ACC/AHA/HRS Guidelines for Device-Based Therapy. *Circulation*. 2008;117:e350–e408.

Does my patient need an implantable-cardioverter-defibrillator (ICD)?

KEY CONCEPT	The decision to place an implantable-cardioverter-defibrillator (ICD) in a patient is based upon cardiac function, conduction abnormalities, and underlying conditions.
HISTORY	HPI: Syncope, palpitations, fatigue, dyspnea, decreased exercise tolerance. PMH: Cardiac arrest, ventricular tachycardia, congestive heart failure, coronary artery disease.
ELECTRO-CARDIOGRAM	Q waves (prior MI), wide QRS complex or BBB.
IMAGING	ECHO: LVEF <40%, LA & LV enlargement, wall motion abnormalities.
SYNTHESIS	**ICD** = Refer patient for placement of **I**mplantable-**C**ardioverter-**D**efibrillator. **SCA** = **S**urvivors of **C**ardiac **A**rrest due to ventricular fibrillation or hemodynamically unstable sustained VT after evaluation to define the cause of the event and to exclude any completely reversible causes. **SHD** = Patients with **S**tructural **H**eart **D**isease and spontaneous sustained VT, whether hemodynamically stable or unstable. **SYNC** = Patients with **SYNC**ope of undetermined origin with clinically relevant, hemodynamically significant sustained VT or ventricular fibrillation induced at electrophysiological study. **PRMI-EF35** = Patients with LVEF <35% due to **PR**ior **M**yocardial **I**nfarction who are at least 40 days post-myocardial infarction and are in NYHA functional Class II or III. **NIDC** = Patients with **N**on**I**schemic **D**ilated **C**ardiomyopathy who have an LVEF ≤35% and who are in NYHA functional Class II or III. **LVDF** = Patients with **LV** **D**ys**F**unction due to prior myocardial infarction who are at least 40 days post-myocardial infarction, have an LVEF <30%, and are in NYHA functional Class I. **NSVT-PRMI** = Patients with **N**on**S**ustained **VT** due to **PR**ior **M**yocardial **I**nfarction, LVEF <40%, and inducible ventricular fibrillation or sustained VT at electrophysiological study.
E **EPIPHANY**	**SCA = ICD** **SHD = ICD** **SYNC = ICD** **PRMI-EF35 = ICD** **NIDC = ICD** **LVDF = ICD** **NSVT-PRMI = ICD**

 DISCUSSION	In survivors of sudden cardiac arrest and those at risk, prevention of a recurrent arrest is the central goal of long-term management. ICDs are the preferred approach as this can treat a ventricular arrhythmia promptly.
 PEARLS	The energy of the first shock by the ICD is set at least 10 J above the threshold of the last defibrillation measured.
 REFERENCE	1) Epstein, et al. ACC/AHA/HRS 2008 Guidelines for Device Based Therapy of Cardiac Rhythm Abnormalities. *J Am Coll Cardiol.* 2008;51:2085–2105. 2) Dimarco JP. Implantable cardioverter-defibrillators. *N Engl J Med.* 2003; 349:1836–1847.

Does my patient need further evaluation with cardiac computed tomography?

KEY CONCEPT	The decision to send a patient for cardiac computed tomography (CCT) is based upon the need for further assessment of cardiac structure and function.
HISTORY	HPI: Patient undergoing CCT for cardiac evaluation. PMH: Coronary artery disease, heart failure, adult congenital heart disease. PSH: Coronary artery bypass graft (CABG), prosthetic valve placement.
SYNTHESIS	**CCT** = Refer patient for **C**ardiac **C**omputed **T**omography. **SYMP-CP** = **SYMP**toms of **C**hest **P**ain, chest tightness, dyspnea, diminished exercise capacity + concern clinically. **ASYMP** = **ASYMP**tomatic. **N-EXER** = **N**ormal **EXER**cise ECG stress test. **P-STR** = **P**ositive **STR**ess imaging test. **N-STR** = **N**ormal **STR**ess imaging test. **NOHF** = **N**ew **O**nset **H**eart **F**ailure with LV systolic dysfunction. **CCS** = **C**oronary **C**alcium Agatston **S**core >100. **G-PAT** = Evaluation of **G**raft **PAT**ency after CABG. **ANOM** = Assessment of **ANOM**alies of coronary arterial and other thoracic arteriovenous vessels. **CHD** = Assessment of complex adult **C**ongenital **H**eart **D**isease. **VALVE** = Evaluation of native and prosthetic cardiac **VALVE**s if clinically suspect significant valvular dysfunction. **MASS** = Evaluation of suspected cardiac **MASS** (tumor or thrombus). **ABL** = Prior to radiofrequency **ABL**ation for atrial fibrillation. **REOP** = Patient undergoing **REOP**erative chest or cardiac surgery.
E **EPIPHANY**	**SYMP = CCT** **N-EXER + SYMP-CP = CCT** **N-STR + SYMP-CP = CCT** **P-STR = CCT** **NOHF = CCT** **CCS = CCT** **G-PAT = CCT** **REOP = CCT** **ANOM = CCT** **CHD = CCT** **VALVE = CCT** **MASS = CCT** **ABL = CCT**

DISCUSSION	The quality of the final image of the CCT is dependent on preparation of the patient and technique by the operator to achieve the highest diagnostic quality that can aid in the assessment of cardiac structure and function.
PEARLS	Patients are optimally suited for cardiac computed tomography under the following conditions: rate at a level commensurate with the temporal resolution of the available scanner, body mass index < 40 kg/m^2, and normal renal function.
REFERENCE	1) Hendel RC, et al. ACCF/ASNC/ACR/AHA/ASE/SCCT/SCMR/SNM 2009 Appropriate Use Criteria for Cardiac Radionuclide Imaging. *Circulation*. 2009;119:e561–e587.

ACS

How do I use a TIMI risk score in the patient with unstable angina/non-ST elevation myocardial infarction (UA/NSTEMI)?

 KEY CONCEPT	The thrombolysis in myocardial infarction (TIMI) risk score is used for prognostication and therapeutic decision making in patients with unstable angina/non-ST elevation MI (UA/NSTEMI).
 HISTORY	HPI: Symptoms of chest pain, dyspnea, diaphoresis. PMH: Coronary artery disease (CAD), prior myocardial infraction (MI), hypertension (HTN), hyperlipidemia, diabetes. FH: Premature CAD or MI. SH: Smoking, alcohol. Labs: Elevated troponin or CKMB.
 ELECTRO-CARDIOGRAM	ST-segment depression of > 0.5 mm in two or more contiguous ECG leads.

SYNTHESIS (cont. on next page)	**UA/NSTEMI** = **U**nstable **A**ngina/**N**on-**ST E**levation **MI**.
	PCI = Refer for **P**ercutaneous **C**oronary **I**ntervention.
	MED-TX = **MED**ical management = oxygen, aspirin, clopidogrel, nitroglycerine, morphine, metoprolol, unfractionated heparin or enoxaparin (see chapter on initial management of US/NSTEMI).
	GP2B3A = **G**lyco**P**rotein IIb/IIIa (**2B3A**) inhibitors = use either of these: Eptifibatide: 180 mcg/kg bolus (maximum 20 mg) IV over 2 minutes, then 2 mcg/kg/min infusion) (maximum 15 mg/hr) for up to 72 hours. Reduce maintenance dose to 1 mcg/kg/min if creatinine clearance <50 mL/min; contraindicated if creatinine clearance <20 mL/min.
	
	Tirofiban: loading infusion: 0.4 mcg/kg/min over 30 minutes, then 0.1 mcg/kg/min infusion for up to 72 hours. Reduce loading and maintenance infusion by 50% in patients with creatinine clearance < 30 mL/min.
	HIGHR = **HIGH R**isk: patients with non-ST-elevated chest pain with one or more of the following characteristics are at a high risk for an adverse cardiovascular event: hemodynamic instability or cardiogenic shock; severe LVD or HF; persistent angina despite medical therapy; new or worsening mitral regurgitation or VSD; or sustained ventricular arrhythmias.
	TIMI = **TIMI** risk score calculated by assigning 1 point for each of the following factors (pneumonic ARCS-ARCS):
	    Age ≥65 years
	    Risk factors ≥3 (HTN, DM, H/lipid, active smoker, FamHx premature CAD = myocardial infarction, coronary revascularization, or sudden death <55 years old [father/1st degree male rel] or <65 years old [female/1st deg rel])

 SYNTHESIS (cont. from previous page)	CAD (known stenosis >=50%) Salicylate, ie, use of aspirin in prior 7 days Angina Recent and severe (>=2 anginal episodes in past 24 hours). Cardiac enzymes elevated (cTnI or CKMB) ST deviation (new or transient) on ECG >=0.5 mm **TIMI LOW** = **TIMI LOW** risk: score between 0 and 2. **TIMI HIGH** = **TIMI HIGH** risk: score between 3 and 7. **SRT** = Refer patient for stress imaging study to evaluate for inducible ischemia. **SRT-POS** = **St**Ress **T**esting **POS**itive: imaging study showing significant reversible ischemia, left ventricular dysfunction, ejection fraction <0.35, or other high risk findings.
E EPIPHANY	**UA/NSTEMI + HIGHR = MED + GP2B3A + PCI** **UA/NSTEMI + TIMI LOW = MED + SRT** **UA/NSTEMI + TIMI LOW + SRT-POS = MED + PCI** **UA/NSTEMI + TIMI HIGH = MED + GP2B3A + PCI**
 DISCUSSION	Patients with a high (3–7) TIMI risk score should be referred for PCI and those with low (0–1) and intermediate (2) should be further evaluated for the degree of myocardial ischemia.
 CONTRA- INDICATIONS	– Patients at initial presentation may not have elevated cardiac serum biomarkers and could have a falsely low TIMI risk score.
 PEARLS	– TIMI risk score can be correlated an increased risk of death, new or recurrent MI, or recurrent at ischemia requiring revascularization at 14 days: **Score** **Risk %** 0–1 4.7 6–7 40.9
 REFERENCE	1) Antman EM, et al. The TIMI Risk Score for Unstable Angina/Non–ST Elevation MI: A Method for Prognostication and Therapeutic Decision Making. *JAMA*. 2000;284(7):835–842. 2) Wright RS, et al. 2011 ACCF/AHA Focused Update of the Guidelines for the Management of Patients with Unstable Angina/Non–ST-Elevation Myocardial Infarction. *Circulation*. 2011;123;2022–2060.

What is my initial management of an unstable angina (UA)/non-ST-elevation myocardial infarction (NSTEMI) patient?

KEY CONCEPT	The initial management of patients presenting with unstable angina (UA) or an acute non-ST-elevation myocardial infarction (NSTEMI) involves assessment through ECG and biomarkers, and rapid triage to early invasive strategy versus conservative (noninvasive) evaluation and medical therapy.
HISTORY	HPI: Chest pain (tightness, squeezing) radiating to left arm with instant onset, dyspnea. PMH: Coronary artery disease, hypertension, diabetes, hyperlipidemia. FH: Coronary artery disease. SH: Smoking, alcohol, drug use.
ELECTRO-CARDIOGRAM	ST-segment depression of >0.5 mm in two or more contiguous ECG leads.
IMAGING	**Stress Echo:** Left ventricular ejection fraction and baseline function. **Radionuclide myocardial perfusion scan:** Detect areas of myocardial perfusion defects and ischemia.
SYNTHESIS (cont. on next page)	**UA/NSTEMI** = Patient with definite or working diagnosis of unstable angina or non-ST-elevation myocardial infarction. **MON = MON**itor: Perform 12-lead ECG. If does not show changes and patient still symptomatic, repeat after 10 minutes. Place patient on telemetry monitoring. Monitor oxygen saturation and use oxygen generously to keep SaO$_2$ > 94%. Send for immediate cardiac biomarkers (cardiac troponin I and creatinine kinase MB) and repeat q8h. **AC = A**nti**C**oagulate. For antiplatelet therapy, immediately give aspirin 325 mg chewed/swallowed. Give clopidogrel 600 mg oral loading dose (if the patient will likely need cardiac bypass surgery this can be held until time of angiography if angiography is performed acutely). Start heparin infusion at 60 units/kg IV bolus followed by 12 units/kg/hr and titrate to keep PTT between 60–90 seconds. **PAIN** = Relieve **PAIN**. If no contraindications, try sublingual **nitroglycerin** 0.4 mg q5 min × 3. If still chest pain, begin nitroglycerin 5 mcg/min IV and titrate up by 5 mcg/min q5 min to max dose of 20 mcg/min. Contraindications to nitroglycerin include right ventricular infarction, patient has taken phosphodiesterase inhibitors (ex. sildenafil) in last 48 hours, or hypotension (SBP <100 mm Hg). Can also use **morphine sulfate**, try 2 mg IV push and re-administer/titrate dose depending on response. **NORM = NORM**alize blood pressure: Nitroglycerin (see PAIN) used for angina will lower the blood pressure. Can also use metoprolol tartrate 5 mg IV q5 min × 3 or 25 mg PO q12h if no contraindications to beta blockers. Do not be overly aggressive with IV medication. If patient is hypotensive see chapter on cardiogenic shock.

SYNTHESIS (cont. from previous page)	**STRAT** = Decide treatment **STRAT**egy: Namely early invasive with PCI versus conservative strategy. See chapter on TIMI risk score and NSTEMI/UA. **MED-TX** = **MED**ical management: In addition to above, patient should have certain medications that have mortality benefit started prior to discharge (not given emergently). Beta blockers such as metoprolol tartrate 25 mg PO bid. ACE inhibitors such as lisinopril 5 mg PO daily. Aspirin should be continued at 81 m PO daily. If patient had a NSTEMI, clopidogrel should be continued at 75 mg PO daily for one year regardless of angiography results.
EPIPHANY	**UA/NSTEMI = MON + AC + PAIN + NORM + STRAT + MED-TX**
DISCUSSION	If an early invasive strategy is likely, prefer ASA + GP2B3A. If conservative likely, use clopidogrel.
PEARLS	– Troponins are more sensitive than CK-MB for the diagnosis of acute STEMI, as more troponin is found in the heart per gram of myocardium.
REFERENCE	1) Wright RS, et al. 2011 ACCF/AHA Focused Update of the Guidelines for the Management of Patients with Unstable Angina/Non–ST-Elevation Myocardial Infarction. *Circulation.* 2011;123;2022–2060.

What is my initial management for an acute ST elevation myocardial infarction (STEMI)?

KEY CONCEPT	The initial management of STEMI patients involves rapid assessment, reducing myocardial oxygen demand, anticoagulation, and of utmost importance- reperfusion.
HISTORY	HPI: Retrosternal chest pain (tightness, squeezing) radiating to left arm with instant onset, dyspnea; symptoms lasting more than 15 minutes. PMH: Coronary artery disease, hypertension, diabetes, hyperlipidemia. FH: Coronary artery disease. SH: Smoking, alcohol, drug use.
ELECTRO-CARDIOGRAM	Early changes ($<=2$ hours): Hyperacute T-waves, ST-segment elevation. Late changes (>2 hours): Q waves.
SYNTHESIS (cont. on next page)	**STEMI** = Patient with definite or working diagnosis of ST-elevation myocardial infarction. **MON = MON**itor: Perform 12-lead ECG. If does not show changes and patient still symptomatic, repeat after 10 minutes. Place patient on telemetry monitoring. Monitor oxygen saturation and use oxygen generously to keep $SaO_2 > 94\%$. Send for immediate cardiac biomarkers (cardiac troponin I and creatinine kinase MB) and repeat q8h. **RPF** = reperfusion. Optimal will be immediate percutaneous coronary intervention (PCI). See chapter on Acute STEMI **RePerF**usion therapy to decide startegy. Except for circumstances immediately life-threatening (ex. severe hypotension or hypoxia), **DO NOT** delay PCI when available for other treatments. **AC = A**nti**C**oagulate. For antiplatelet therapy, immediately give aspirin 325 mg chewed/swallowed. Give clopidogrel 600 mg oral loading dose (if the patient will likely need cardiac bypass surgery this can be held until time of angiography if angiography is performed acutely). Start heparin infusion at 60 units/kg IV bolus followed by 12 units/kg/hr and titrate to keep PTT between 60–90 seconds. **PAIN** = Relieve **PAIN**. If no contraindications, try sublingual **nitroglycerin** 0.4 mg q5 min × 3. If still chest pain, begin nitroglycerin 5 mcg/min IV and titrate up by 5 mcg/min q5 min to max dose of 20 mcg/min. Contraindications to nitroglycerin include right ventricular infarcton, patient has taken phosphodiesterase inhibitors (ex. sildenafil) in last 48 hours, or hypotension (SBP < 100 mm Hg). Can also use **morphine sulfate**, try 2 mg IV push and re-administer/titrate dose depending on response. **NORM = NORM**alize blood pressure: Nitroglycerin (see PAIN) used for angina will lower the blood pressure. Can also use metoprolol tartrate 5 mg IV q5 min × 3 or 25 mg PO q12h if no contraindications to beta blockers. Do not be overly aggressive with IV medication. If patient is hypotensive see chapter on cardiogenic shock.

SYNTHESIS (cont. from previous page)	**MED-TX = MED**ical management: In addition to above, patient should have certain medications that have mortality benefit started prior to discharge (not given emergently). Beta blockers such as metoprolol tartrate 25 mg PO bid. ACE inhibitors such as lisinopril 5 mg PO daily. Aspirin should be continued at 81 m PO daily. Clopidogrel should be continued at 75 mg PO daily.
EPIPHANY	**STEMI = MON + RPF + AC + PAIN + NORM + MED-TX**
DISCUSSION	The main intervention that changes outcome in STEMI is opening the artery. If PCI becomes available, it should take precedence on the next intervention to be done unless there is an immediate life-threatening circumstance.
PEARLS	– Troponins are more sensitive than CK-MB for the diagnosis of acute STEMI as more troponin is found in the heart per gram of myocardium.
REFERENCE	1) Antman EM, et al. 2007 Focused Update of the ACC/AHA 2004 Guidelines for the Management of Patients with ST-Elevation Myocardial Infarction. *J Am Coll Cardiol.* 2008;51;210–247.

What initial reperfusion strategy should I begin in my patient with an acute STEMI?

 KEY CONCEPT	The reperfusion strategy for an acute ST-Elevation myocardial infarction (STEMI) is based on whether or not PCI is available and contraindications to fibrinolytic therapy.
 HISTORY	HPI: Retrosternal chest pain (tightness, squeezing) radiating to left arm with instant onset, dyspnea, symptoms lasting more than 15 minutes. PMH: Coronary artery disease, hypertension, diabetes, hyperlipidemia. FH: Coronary artery disease. SH: Smoking, alcohol, drug use.
 ELECTRO-CARDIOGRAM	Early changes (< = 2 hours): Hyperacute T-waves, ST-segment elevation Late changes (>2 hours): Q waves.
 SYNTHESIS	**STEMI** = Patient with definite or working diagnosis of acute ST-elevation myocardial infarction <12 hours in duration. See chapter on initial management for **STEMI**. **PCI-90** = **P**ercutaneous **C**oronary **I**ntervention can be performed in **90** minutes or less from time of first medical contact. **PCI-UNAV** = **PCI** is **UNAV**ailable or cannot be done within 90 minutes of first medical contact. **PCI** = Send patient for immediate **P**ercutaneous **C**oronary **I**ntervention. **FIBR** = **FIB**rinolytic therapy: DO NOT give to patient with absolute contraindications (see contraindications box). Options available: Streptokinase 1.5 million units IV over 60 minutes OR Alteplase, IV bolus 15 mg, infusion 0.75 mg/kg over 30 min (maximum 50 mg), then 0.5 mg/kg (maximum 35 mg) over the next 60 min to an overall maximum of 100 mg OR Reteplase, 10 U IV over 2 min, then 30 min later, give 10 U IV over 2 min. OR Tenecteplase, IV bolus over 15 seconds: 30 mg for weight < 60 kg; 35 mg (60–69 kg); 40 mg (70–79 kg); 45 mg (80–89 kg); 50 mg (> =90 kg). **TX-PAT** = **T**ransfer **PAT**ient: Transfer patient as soon as possible to a facility with interventional cardiology for a higher level of care.
E EPIPHANY	**STEMI + PCI-90 = PCI** **STEMI + PCI-UNAV = FIBR + TX-PAT**

DISCUSSION	See chapter on initial management for STEMI for all patients. The main intervention that changes outcome in STEMI is opening the artery. Mechanical reperfusion is superior to chemical reperfusion. If PCI becomes available, it should take precedence as the next intervention to be done unless there is an immediate life-threatening circumstance.
PEARLS	– PCI compared to fibrinolytic therapy has shown enhanced survival and lower rates of intracranial hemorrhage and recurrent MI.
CONTRA-INDICATIONS	Fibrinolytic therapy is **absolutely** contraindicated in patients if previous intracranial hemorrhage, known cerebral vascular lesion/malignant intracranial neoplasm, ischemic stroke/significant closed head/facial trauma in past 3 months, suspected aortic dissection, active bleeding, or bleeding diathesis.
REFERENCE	1) Antman EM, et al. 2007 Focused Update of the ACC/AHA 2004 Guidelines for the Management of Patients with ST-Elevation Myocardial Infarction. *J Am Coll Cardiol.* 2008;51;210–247. 2) Keeley EC. Primary PCI for Myocardial Infarction with ST-Segment Elevation. *N Engl J Med.* 2007;356:47–54.

How do you manage a patient post-MI and treat the complications of MI?

KEY CONCEPT	Patients post-STEMI can have a wide range of serious complications in the 24–48 hour time range.
HISTORY	HPI: Patient with STEMI s/p fibrinolytic or PCI. PMH/PSH: Prior angina or MI, CAD PVD Prior interventions SH: Smoking history, advanced age >70 years. Labs: Biomarker elevation, electrolyte abnormality Inflammatory markers Leukocyte count (greater necrosis), electrolytes for renal perfusion and cardiac output.
PHYSICAL EXAM	Exam: Systolic impulse, new murmurs, JVD, breathing pattern, pulses (weak or bounding), rubs, gallops.
IMAGING	ECG: Recurrent ST elevations, PR depressions (pericarditis?) Arrhythmias/blocks? ECHO: LV function.

SYNTHESIS (cont. on next page)	**RI** = **R**ecurrent **I**schemia.
	EMT = **E**scalate **M**edical **T**herapy and correct secondary causes of ischemia.
	IABP = **IABP** if hemodynamic instability/poor LV function, or large area of myocardium at risk.
	CATH = Obtain ECG. If no ST elevation and ischemia not controlled, then refer for **CATH**eterization; if ischemia controlled, then nonurgent PCI or CABG.
	FIBRIN = If ST elevation, then **FIBRIN**olytic therapy or PCI based on availability/contraindications.
	PULMC = **PULM**onary **C**ongestion.
	FOM = **F**urosemide 0.5 mg/kg, **O**xygen, **M**orphine.
	NITRO = **NITRO**glycerin 10–20 mcg/min if SBP >100.
	PRESSOR = Dopamine, dobutamine—check blood pressure and if >100 and not less than 30 below baseline, then start ACEI.
	       SPB>100, give nitroglycerin 10–20 mcg/min
	       SBP 70–100 and no shock, give dobutamine 2–20 mcg/kg/min
	       SBP 70–100 with shock, give dopamine 5–15 mcg/kg/min
	       SBP <70 with shock, give norepinephrine 0.5–30 mcg/min
	HYPO = **HYPO**volemia/**HYPO**tension.
	F = **F**luids.
	B = **B**lood **D** = **D**iuretics **N** = **N**itrates **BB** = **B**eta **B**lockers.
	ACEI = **ACE**-Inhibitors **HTN** = **H**yper**T**ensio**N** **CCB** = **C**al**C**ium **B**lockers.
	DIG = **DIG**oxin **ASA** = Aspirin/NSAID **SWAN** = Place **SWAN**-Ganz and monitor wedge pressure **ADEN** = **ADEN**osine **CV** = **C**ardio**V**ersion.
	CS = **C**ardiogenic **S**hock **A** = **A**rrhythmia **BRAD** = **BRAD**ycardia.
	ATRO = **ATRO**pine (caution if unstable, may worsen ischemia with increased HR, pacemaker for heart blocks) **SVT** = **S**upra**V**entricular **T**achycardia **VTF** = **V**entricular **T**achycardia, **F**ibrillation.

SYNTHESIS (cont. from previous page)	**PM** = **P**ace**M**aker **RVI** = **RV** Infarction **PMR** = **P**apillary **M**uscle **R**upture **SURG** = Urgent **SURG**ical Repair **VSR** = **V**entricle **S**eptal **R**upture **LV** = LVFWR free wall rupture **P** = **P**ericarditis.
E EPIPHANY	**RI = EMT + IABP ± CATH ± FIBRIN** **PULMC = FOM ± NITRO/PRESSOR** **HYPO = F + B + PRESSOR + IABP** **HTN = N + D + BB + ACEI** **CS = SWAN + N + PRESSOR + IABP ± FIBRIN ± CATH** **A + BRAD = ATRO** **A + SVT = BB or DIG or ADEN or CCB or CV** **A + VFT = EMT + CV or BB or AMIO or PM** **RVI = F+ PRESSOR** **PMR = IABP + PRESSOR + SURG** **VSR = IABP + PRESSOR + SURG** **LVFWR = SURG** **P = ASA**
DISCUSSION	Any new systolic murmur post-MI is likely VSD versus MR. Increased risk of mortality, reinfarction, hypertension, heart failure, and myocardial rupture associated with NSAID (except ASA). Avoid beta blockers if heart failure, low output state, heart block, asthma, reactive airway disease.
PEARLS	IAPB is used in STEMI patients with hypotension < 90 or 30 mm Hg below baseline who do not respond to other interventions, low output state, cardiogenic shock not quickly reversed, recurrent ischemic pain, and hemodynamic instability/poor LV function, large myocardial risk.
REFERENCE	1) Antman EM, et al. ACC/AHA Guidelines for the Management of Patients with ST Elevation Myocardial Infarction. *Circulation.* 2004 Aug 21;110 (9):282–292. 2) Antman EM, et al. 2007 Focused Update of the ACC/AHA 2004 Guidelines for the Management of Patients with ST Elevation Myocardial Infarction. *J Am Coll Cardiol.* 2008 Jan 15;51(2):210–247.

How do I manage variant angina?

 KEY CONCEPT	The management of variant angina (VA) is based upon risk factor modification, medical therapy to relieve coronary vasospasm, and percutaneous coronary intervention (PCI) if necessary.
 HISTORY	HPI: Sudden onset of chest pain at rest usually occurring in the early morning. PMH: Coronary artery disease, hypertension, hyperlipidemia, diabetes, Raynaud's phenomenon. SH: Smoking, alcohol, cocaine use.
 ELECTRO-CARDIOGRAM	ST-elevation with return to baseline upon resolution of symptoms.
 IMAGING	**Coronary angiography:** Administration of ergonovine can provoke coronary artery vasospasm, which in the affected coronary artery will result in an initial increase in flow, followed by an abrupt decrease in flow. In normal coronary arteries, the luminal reduction is mild and diffuse with no change in flow velocity.
 SYNTHESIS	**CAD** = **C**oronary **A**rtery **D**isease. **DILT** = **DILT**iazem 240 mg/day. **INEFF-DILT** = **DILT**iazem is **INEFF**ective. **NIT** = Sublingual isosorbide di**NIT**rate 5 mg Q5 minutes, maximum dose 15 mg. **PCI** = **P**ercutaneous **C**oronary **I**ntervention. **RFM** = **R**isk **F**actor **M**odification: smoking cessation, blood pressure control (see chapter on hypertension), lipid management (see chapter on LDL management), weight management. **VARANG** = patient diagnosed with **VAR**iant **ANG**ina. **VARANG-REF** = **V**ariant **A**ngina **R**efractory to medical therapy.
E EPIPHANY	**VARANG = RFM + DILT** **VARANG + INEFF-DILT = NIT** **VARANG-REF + CAD = PCI**
 DISCUSSION	Risk factor modification is important in the long-term management of variant angina. Smoking, hypertension, and hyperlipidemia all contribute to endothelial dysfunction, which can cause coronary vasospasm.

 CONTRA- INDICATIONS	– Nonselective beta blockers such as propanolol should be avoided in patients with VA as it can further exacerbate coronary vasospasm. – Aspirin should be avoided in patients with VA as it inhibits the production of prostacyclin, a vasodilator. – PCI is contraindicated in patients with an acute spasm and minimally obstructive disease.
 PEARLS	– Patients with variant angina receiving medical therapy with near-to-normal coronary arteries have a 95% 5-year survival rate. – Patients with variant angina receiving medical therapy with multivessel disease have an 80% 5-year survival rate.
 REFERENCE	1) Anderson JL, et al. ACC/AHA 2007 Guidelines on Perioperative Cardiovascular Evaluation and Care for Noncardiac Surgery: Executive Summary. *J Am Coll Cardiol.* 2007;50:e1–e157.

Should I refer my patient for PCI or CABG?

 KEY CONCEPT	Coronary-artery bypass graft (CABG) is indicated for severe coronary artery disease when the benefits of survival and quality of life (symptoms and functional status) exceed the consequences and morbidity of surgery.
 HISTORY	HPI: Patient with coronary artery disease (CAD) who is in need of coronary revascularization. PMH: CAD, hypertension, hyperlipidemia, diabetes, myocardial infarction, angina, heart failure. PSH: CABG, percutaneous coronary intervention (angioplasty). SH: Smoking, alcohol, illicit drug use.
 ELECTRO-CARDIOGRAM	ST-elevation, ST-depression, deep Q waves (>1 mm), poor R-wave progression.
 IMAGING	**Stress Echo:** Left ventricular ejection fraction and baseline function. **Radionuclide myocardial perfusion scan:** Detect areas of myocardial perfusion defects and ischemia.
 SYNTHESIS	**CABG** = Send patient for **CABG**. **PCI** = Send patient for percutaneous intervention. **LMD** = **L**eft **M**ain **D**isease = >50% stenosis in left main coronary artery. **1VD** = **1 V**essel **D**isease = >70% stenosis in 1 non-left main coronary artery vessel **2VD** = **2 V**essel **D**isease = >70% stenosis 2 non-left main coronary artery vessels. **3VD** = **3 V**essel **D**isease = >70% stenosis in 3 non-left main coronary artery vessels. **PROX-LAD** = **PROX**imal **LAD** stenosis = >70% stenosis in proximal left anterior descending artery. **DM** = **D**iabetes **M**ellitis. **ISCH** = **ISCH**emia on noninvasive testing. **LVEF-50** = **L**eft **V**entricular **E**jection **F**raction <50%. **LIMA** = **L**eft **I**nternal **M**ammary **A**rtery.
E EPIPHANY	1VD = PCI 2VD = PCI 2VD + PROX-LAD + DM = CABG 2VD + LVEF-50 = CABG 2VD + ISCH = CABG 3VD = CABG LMD = CABG
 DISCUSSION	CABG is indicated over PCI in patients with left main and multivessel disease with the presence of diabetes, left ventricular dysfunction, and significant areas of myocardial ischemia. All patients will need aggressive risk factor modification post intervention.

CONTRA-INDICATIONS	– There are no studies comparing efficacy of CABG to placebo – Left main artery lesions are the most dangerous and become the most unstable after cardiac catheterization and are not safe for angioplasty.
PEARLS	– Grafts usually last 10–15 years. – CABG has been shown to have lower-rate major adverse cardiac or cerebrovascular events compared to PCI in patients with left main or 3 vessel disease. – Patients treated with CABG versus DES have lower rates of death or MI in multivessel disease and have lower rates of revascularization.
REFERENCE	1) Hannan EL, et al. Drug-Eluting Stents vs. Coronary-Artery Bypass. *N Engl J Med.* 2008;358(4):331–341. 2) Patel MR, et al. Appropriateness Criteria for Coronary Revascularization. *Circulation.* 2009;119:1330–1352. 3) Serruys P, et al. Percutaneous Coronary Intervention versus Coronary Artery Bypass Grafting for Severe Coronary Artery Disease. *N Engl J Med.* 2009;360:961–972.

How do I determine the site of STEMI infarct/injury on ECG?

KEY CONCEPT	It is important to understand the location of infarct and injury to aid in management decisions. Certain areas of infarction will manifest in different leads on the ECG.
HISTORY	Patient presents with chest pain and palpitations.
ELECTRO-CARDIOGRAM	Anteroseptal (V1-3) Anterolatertal (V3-6, I, aVL) Lateral (I, aVL, V5, V6) Inferior (II, III, aVF) Posterior (V1-3 mirror image)
SYNTHESIS	**STEMI** = ST segment elevation. **SD** = ST **S**egment **D**epression **LM** = **L**eft **M**ain occlusion. **D-LAD** = **D**istal **LAD**. **P-LAD** = **P**roximal **LAD**. **LAT** = **LAT**eral. **POST** = **POST**erior. **CIRC** = **CIRC**umflex. **RCA** = **R**ight **C**oronary. **Q** = **Q** wave location in patient with STEMI. **INF** = **INF**erior. **RV** = **R**ight **V**entricular. **ANT** = **ANT**erior. **POST** = **POST**erior. **AP** = Antero-septal.
EPIPHANY	**STEMI:** **LM = STEMI in aVR, V1, ST depression in II, aVF, v-V6** **D-LAD = STEMI in V3-V6, II, ST depression in aVR** **P-LAD = STEMI in aVR, aVL, V1-V4, St depression in II, III, aVF** **LAT = STEMI in I, aVL, V5-V6** **POST = SD in V1-V3** **CIRC = STEMI in II/III** **RCA = STEMI in III/II, SD in I, positive T wave in V4R** **Q/Infarct:** **INF = Q in II/III/aVF** **RV = Q in V4R-V6R** **ANT = Q in V3-V4** **POST = Q in V1** **AP = Q in V1-V3**

DISCUSSION	Knowing the blood supply can aid in diagnosis: – The LAD supplies the anterior wall and interventricular septum. – The RCA supplies the inferior wall and sinus and AV node. Occlusion results in inferior MI, sinus bradycardia and heart blocks. Occlusion of the left main coronary leads to anterior MI, pump failure and sudden death. Occlusion of the LAD causes anterior MI, LV failure, arrhythmias, and blocks. Occlusion of the left circumflex leads to lateral infarcts.
PEARLS	Obtain ECG during episodes of chest pain because the findings may be transient. The progression of STEMI is hyperacute T waves to ST elevation to abnormal Q waves to T wave inversion. If possible compare prior ECG to determine if abnormalities are new or old. Q waves can also be seen in sarcoid, amyloid, tumor, scleroderma, and myocardial inflammation.
REFERENCE	1) Wellens HJJ, Conover M. *The ECG in Emergency Decision Making.* 2nd ed. St. Louis, MO: Saunders, Elsevier; 2006. 2) Wagner GS. Marriotts *Practical Electrocardiography.* 10th ed. New York, NY: Lippincott Williams and Wilkins; 2000.

How do I manage a patient with right/inferior myocardial infarction?

 KEY CONCEPT	The management of right ventricular myocardial infarction includes special considerations compared with classic left ventricular infarctions.
 HISTORY	Indigestion, nausea, vomiting, diaphoresis, lightheadedness, chest pain.
 PHYSICAL EXAM	Hypotension, bradycardia, distended neck veins/elevated jugular venous pressure (increased during inspiration), prominent A or V waves of venous pulse, clear lung fields, right-sided S3/4 gallops, tricuspid regurgitation, pulsus paradoxus, cardiogenic shock.
 ELECTRO-CARDIOGRAM	Often there is evidence of inferior wall myocardial infarction on a standard ECG. Obtain right side ECG to evaluate right ventricle. ST elevation in II, III, aVF (III > II see "determine the site of infarct on ECG" chapter) Reciprocal St depression in I, aVL ST elevation in V4R-V6R 1st or 2nd degree AV block
 IMAGING	CXR: Pulmonary edema may be absent. ECHO: Tricuspid regurgitation, regional RV wall motion abnormalities, dilated RV, decreased ejection fraction. Swanz: Elevated right atrial pressures > 10 mm Hg, low pulmonary systolic pressures, low wedge pressure.
 SYNTHESIS	**R-MI** = Patient with definite or working diagnosis of acute **R**ight ventricular **M**yocardial **I**nfarction. **HU** = **H**emodynamically **U**nstable: hypotension (systolic BP < 90 mm Hg), significant bradycardia (ventricular rate < 55 bpm or periods of asystole > 3 seconds), or evidence of shock (mental status changes or decreased urine output). **HS** = **H**emodynamically **S**table: normotensive, normal mentation, no evidence of shock. **STAB** = **STAB**ilize. Give IV fluids wide open if hypotensive. If inadequate response, start dopamine infusion at 5 mcg/kg/min and titrate to MAP > 60 mm Hg. See chapter on cardiogenic shock. For bradycardia, can try atropine 1 mg IV. Often dopamine will increase heart rate as well. If still bradycardic can use temporary pacing with transcutaneous pacing pads or transvenous pacemaker. **MI-TX:** See chapter on STEMI for instruction on anticoagulation, monitoring, and reperfusion. **MED-TX:** Special considerations: beta blockers may be counterproductive as they worsen bradycardia. Patients are preload dependent- nitrates and diuretics can cause severe hypotension. If mechanical ventilation is required, a strategy with lower PEEP is often used.

EPIPHANY	**R-MI + HS = MI-TX + MED-TX** **R-MI + HU = STAB + MI-TX + MED-TX**
DISCUSSION	Up to 50% of patients with inferior MI also have RV involvement; however, only 10% of patients have hemodynamically significant RV dysfunction. Patients will need volume to increase left heart filling to restore cardiac output and sustain perfusion. Bradyarrhythmias are more common in inferior MI from increased vagal tone and possible SA node involvement. The SA node is supplied by the RCA.
PEARLS	Do not give nitrates or diuretics (will cause reduction of preload and further hypotension). Do not confuse presentation with CHF, if the patient has worsening hypotension; then consider RV infarction. RV infarcts may be difficult to distinguish from CHF, PE, and tamponade.
REFERENCE	1) Goldstein JA. Pathophysiology and Management of Right Heart Ischemia. *J Am Coll Cardio.* 2002;40:841. 2) Isner JM. Right Ventricular Myocardial infarction. *JAMA.* 1988;259:712. 3) Kinch JW, Ryan TJ. Right Ventricular Infarction. *N Eng J Med.* 1994;330:1211.

How to manage a patient with elevated troponins?

KEY CONCEPT	Troponins (Tc, Ti, Tt) are biomarkers used to assess myocardial injury that have become important for diagnosis of MI/NSTEMI when symptoms and ECG abnormalities are nonspecific or absent. Troponins are positive when >0.04; levels are undetectable in most normal subjects. Tc is not used clinically.
HISTORY	HPI: Chest pain (quality, type, location, duration, aggravating/relieving factors, intensity), any recent viral infections—myocarditis, any chest trauma check for pericardial tamponade, recent chemotherapy that is cardiotoxic. PE: Assess vitals for high temperature (sepsis/SIRS), blood pressure for volume status (dry mucous membranes, low JVP, low CVP), or hypertensive emergency with organ damage. Labs: BUN/creatinine for renal failure, hemoglobin to asses for anemia or workup for GI bleed, UDS-look for cocaine. PM Hx/PSx Hx: CAD (history of MI, CABG, angioplasty, angina) CHF (prior low EF, hx of AICD implant. Social/Fhx: Drug use.
ELECTRO-CARDIOGRAM	ECG: ST depression.
SYNTHESIS	**CLIN-ACS = CLIN**ical **ACS**: patient presents with a good clinical picture for ACS, ie, positive history and ECG. **CLIN-OT = CLIN**ical **OT**her: patient presents with a good clinical picture for ACS, but there are other important conditions present that may have precipitated the clinical presentation and need to be addressed promptly, eg, an acute gastrointestinal bleed, severe anemia, supraventricular or ventricular tachycardia, pulmonary embolism. **CKMBNL = CKMB** levels **N**ormal making one suspect an alternative diagnosis for the elevated troponin level (normal CKMB will rise in parallel with troponins). **CKMBEL = CKMB** levels abnormally **EL**evated. **TROP-POS = TROP**onin **POS**itive. **ACS** = Likely **ACS** (refer to ACS chapter for further management). **NON-ACS** = A **NON-ACS** case, with elevated troponins likely secondary to another clinical condition such as heart failure, sepsis, pulmonary emboli. **ISBURD = IS**chemic **BURD**en evaluation should be considered once the other clinical issues have been diagnoses and managed appropriately.
EPIPHANY	**CLIN-ACS + TROP-POS = ACS** **CLIN-OT + TROP-POS + CKMBNL = NON-ACS** **CLIN-OT + TROP-POS + CKMBEL = ISBURD**

DISCUSSION	Elevated troponins are not necessarily due to ACS. Troponins can be released in conditions that cause membrane permeability/demand ischemia (mismatch between oxygen supply and demand). The most common causes in patients with normal angiogram included tachycardia 28%, pericarditis10%, heart failure 5%, strenuous exercise 10%, and no clear precipitating event 47%. Elevations in the normal population are rare without coexisting renal failure, diabetes, LVH, and heart failure.
PEARLS	Troponin elevations are nonspecific in patient with low pretest probability of ACS, and thus may divert attention from the underlying clinical problem. Troponins are sensitive to rule out NSTEMI but less specific to rule in NSTEMI.
REFERENCE	1) Higgins JP, et al. Elevation of Cardiac Troponin I Indicates More Than Myocardial Ischemia. *Clin Invest Med.* 2003;26(3):133–147.

How do I manage a patient with chronic stable angina?

KEY CONCEPT	Angina is characterized by chest pain caused by inability of oxygen supply to meet demand. It is the initial manifestation of CAD in close to 50% of patients.

HISTORY	HPI: Patient presents with chest pain.
	Canadian Cardiovascular Society Classification Angina Grading:
	    1—symptoms with marked exertion
	    2—slight limitation of ordinary activity
	    3—marked limitation of activity
	    4—inability to carry out physical activity
	PMH: CAD, MI, hypertension, hyperlipidemia.
	SH: Smoking use, alcohol intake.
	FH: Premature CAD/MI, PVD/CVD.

ELECTRO-CARDIOGRAM	ECG: ST depression, transient ST elevations.
SYNTHESIS (cont. on next page)	**CSA = C**hronic **S**table **A**ngina: characterized by substernal location, provoked by exertion or stress, and relived by rest or nitroglycerine. **FHR = F**eatures of **H**igh **R**isk: pain lasting >20 minutes, age >65 years, ST and T wave changes, pulmonary edema, symptoms refractory to therapy. **CST-POS = C**ardiac **S**tress **T**est **POS**itive: if moderate pretest probability for CAD and stable symptoms, then stress ECG testing. **CATH = C**ardiac **CATH**eterization. **TRC = T**reat **R**eversible **C**auses, eg, hypertension, hyperlipidemia (target LDL <100), CHF, anemia, hypoxemia, glucose control, drug side effect, thyroid disease. Goal Blood pressures: <140/90 mm Hg Most adults with hypertension <130/80 mm Hg Diabetes, chronic kidney disease, known CAD, CAD equivalents (carotid artery disease [carotid bruit, or abnormal carotid ultrasound/angiography], AAA & PVD), or 10-year Framingham risk score of >/=10% <120/80 mm Hg Left ventricular dysfunction (ejection fraction <40%) **NTG = **Use nitroglycerine 0.4 mg SL q5 min × 3 prn (can use prophylactically). **LAN = L**ong **A**cting **N**itrate preparations. **ASA = A**spirin (if no contraindications) 81 mg orally each day. **BB = B**eta **B**lockers (atenolol, metoprolol) to reduce symptoms (caution in Printzmetal angina).

 SYNTHESIS (cont. from previous page)	**CCB** = **C**alcium **C**hannel **B**lockers (amlodipine, nifedipine) for coronary vasodilation (indicated for Printzmetal angina). **ACEI** = **A**ngiotensin **C**onverting **E**nzyme **I**nhibitors = in patients with diabetes or LV systolic dysfunction, LVEF <40%. **DIET** = **DIET** modification (reduced cholesterol, fat). **EXER** = **EXER**cise program.
 EPIPHANY	**CSA = TRC + NTG + LAN + ASA + BB/CCB + ACEI + DIET + EXER** **FHR = CATH** **CST-POS = CATH**
 DISCUSSION	Significant CAD is stenosis >70% if one major epicardial artery or 50% of LAD. The goal of treatment is to reduce ischemia and risk factors for coronary artery disease. The subendocardial layer is most vulnerable to ischemia and receives blood during diastole. Medical therapy aims at increasing coronary blood supply, decreasing myocardial oxygen demand, and stabilization of vulnerable plaques. Patients with left main, three-vessel, or two-vessel CAD with significant stenosis of the proximal LAD may have a survival advantage with revascularization. Low-risk patients with chronic stable angina should be treated with medical therapy prior to any intervention.
 PEARLS	Nitroglyercine should be renewed every 3–6 months; allow intervals of 8–10 hours to avoid tolerance. Percutaneous coronary intervention provides better symptomatic relief than medical therapy but does not decrease future risk of MI or death.
 REFERENCE	1) Gibbons RJ, et al. ACC/AHA 2002 Guideline Update for the Management of Patients with Chronic Stable Angina. *Circulation* 2002. 2) Rosendorff C, et al. Treatment of Hypertension in the Prevention and Management of Ischemic Heart Disease. *Circulation.* 2007;115(21):2761–2788.

Should our patient get an intra-aortic balloon pump placed?

KEY CONCEPT	Intra-aortic balloon pump (IABP) counterpulsation is a circulatory assist technique with use in certain clinical settings.
HISTORY	Patient presents with ACS and may have high risk features: age >70, EF <45, suboptimal PTCA results, presence of arrhythmias, three vessel disease, hemodynamic instability.
PHYSICAL EXAM	CV: Hypotension, weak diminished pulses, murmur of MR/AS. Resp: Pulmonary crackles.
ELECTRO-CARDIOGRAM	Does the patient have ventricular tachycardia/fibrillation that causes hemodynamic instability?
IMAGING	ECHO: Determine if mitral regurgitation (papillary muscle rupture or ventricular septal rupture). Determine if depressed LVEF or cardiogenic shock. CXR: Pulmonary congestion.
SYNTHESIS	**IABP** = Refer for intra-aortic balloon pump (**IABP**) counterpulsation. **CI-IABP** = **C**ontra**I**ndication to **I**ntra**A**ortic **B**alloon **P**ump: 1) AR or AV shunting 2) AAA or aortic dissection 3) Sepsis 4) Bleeding disorder 5) Bilateral PVD/femoral popliteal bypass grafts **NO-CI-IABP** = **NO CI-IABP**. **CG-SHOCK** = **C**ardio**G**enic **SHOCK** (SBP <90 mm Hg or 30 mm Hg below baseline) not amenable by pressors/inotropes. **SPT-HIGHR** = **S**u**P**por**T** for **HIGH-R**isk catheterization/percutaneous coronary intervention/cardiac surgery. **ACS-SEV-ISCH** = **ACS** patients (UA/NSTEMI/STEMI) with continuing **SEV**ere **ISCH**emia despite intensive medical therapy. **AMI-HIGHR** = **A**cute **M**yocardial **I**nfarction patients who are severely ill and thus at **HIGH R**isk and undergoing acute myocardial revascularization (cardiac catheterization, percutaneous coronary intervention, surgical revascularization). **AMI-MECO** = **A**cute **M**yocardial **I**nfarction with **ME**chanical **CO**mplications (ventricular septal defect, papillary muscle rupture/severe mitral regurgitation). **REFRAC AN-HF-VA** = Patient with **REFRAC**tory **A**ngina/**H**eart **F**ailure/**V**entricular **A**rrhythmias despite medical therapy. **WEAN-CPB** = Patient needing assistance on **WEAN**ing from **C**ardio**P**ulmonary **B**ypass.

 EPIPHANY	**CG-SHOCK + NO-CI-IABP = IABP** **SPT-HIGHR + NO-CI-IABP = IABP** **ACS-SEV-ISCH + NO-CI-IABP = IABP** **AMI-HIGHR + NO-CI-IABP = IABP** **AMI-MECO + NO-CI-IABP = IABP** **REFRAC AN-HF-VA + NO-CI-IABP = IABP** **WEAN-CPB + NO-CI-IABP = IABP**
 DISCUSSION	During diastole, blood is displaced to proximal aorta via inflation to aid in coronary blood flow. During systole, afterload and myocardial oxygen consumption are reduced by a vacuum effect created by deflation.
 PEARLS	Use of IABP is beneficial for hemodynamic support and stabilization during high-risk angiography and revascularization. Note factors that can increase complication rate include PVD, age >70, female sex, diabetes/HTN, prolonged support, large catheter/large body surface area. Complications include limb ischemia, bleeding, balloon leak, IABP failure, arterial dissection.
 REFERENCE	1) Stone GW, et al. Contemporary Utilization and Outcomes of Intra-aortic Balloon Counterpulsation in Acute Myocardial Infarction: The Benchmark Registry. *J Am Coll Cardiol.* 2003;41:1940–1945. 2) Antman EM, et al. 2007 Focused Update of the ACC/AHA 2004 Guidelines for the Management of Patients With ST-Elevation Myocardial Infarction. *J Am Coll Cardiol.* 2008;51;210–247. 3) Wright RS, et al. 2011 ACCF/AHA Focused Update of the Guidelines for the Management of Patients with Unstable Angina/Non–ST-Elevation Myocardial Infarction. *Circulation.* 2011;123;2022–2060.

How do I manage a patient presenting with cocaine-induced chest pain?

KEY CONCEPT	Cocaine is a drug of abuse that causes myocardial ischemia through coronary artery spasm.
HISTORY	HPI: Patient presenting with chest pain, palpitations, dyspnea, anxiety. SH: Drug use, smoking, alcohol. Labs: Urine drug screen positive for cocaine, positive cardiac biomarkers.
PHYSICAL EXAM	Elevated blood pressure, tachycardia.
ELECTRO-CARDIOGRAM	ST elevation, widened QRS, QT-c prolongation.
SYNTHESIS	**CICP** = **C**ocaine-**I**nduced **C**hest **P**ain. **1STLT** = **1ST** **L**ine **T**herapy: aspirin, nitroglycerine, oxygen (see chapter on UA/NSTEMI) and in addition give lorazepam 1 mg IV every 5 minutes (max 8 mg); or diazepam 5–10 mg IV, then 5 mg IV every 20 minutes (max 20 mg). **2NDLT** = **2ND** **L**ine **T**herapy: phentolamine (1 mg IV, then 2.5 mg IV q15 minutes until blood pressure controlled) or verapamil 2.5 mg IV over 2 minutes; if no response, give 5 mg every 20 minutes (maximum 20 mg total). **PCI** = Refer for **P**er**C**utaneous **I**ntervention. **NO-PCI** = **NO PCI** facilities available. **TL** = Administer **T**hrombo**L**ytics if no contraindications (see STEMI chapter). **CCP** = **C**ontinuing **C**hest **P**ain. **STEMI** = **ST**-**E**levation **M**yocardial **I**nfarction (see STEMI chapter).

E
EPIPHANY
	Steps in management of patient with cocaine-induced chest pain:
	1) **CICP = 1STLT**
	2) **1SLT + CCP = 2NDLT**
	3) **2NDLT+ CCP = PCI**
	    2NDLT + STEMI = PCI
	    2NDLT + STEMI + NO-PCI = TL

DISCUSSION	The toxic effects of cocaine are caused by the inhibition of norepinephrine reuptake. Myocardial ischemia occurs from cocaine abuse through coronary artery vasospasm. Benzodiazepines decrease central stimulatory effects of cocaine and decrease cardiac toxicity. Phentolamine counteracts alpha-adrenergic effects, and calcium channel blockers are used to counteract vasospasm. Cessation of cocaine use should be advised as recurrent chest pain and MI are less common after discontinuation.

 CONTRA-INDICATIONS	– Beta blockers should be avoided because of the risk of exacerbating coronary vasospasm effect of cocaine. If beta blocker is needed, use with caution, and use labetalol or carvedilol for its alpha blockade effects.
 PEARLS	– If decision is made to place stent, then bare metal stent is preferred. – Majority of cocaine-induced myocardial infarctions occur within 24 hours of use. – Concomitant use of cigarettes with cocaine can exacerbate coronary artery vasoconstriction and further increase myocardial oxygen demand. – Ingestion of ethanol with cocaine produces metabolite cocaethylene, which blocks the reuptake of dopamine in the synaptic cleft and potentiates the toxic effects of cocaine.
REFERENCE	1) McCord J, et al. Management of Cocaine-Associated Chest Pain and Myocardial Infarction. *Circulation.* 2008;117:1897–1907. 2) Lange RA, et al. Cardiovascular Complications of Cocaine Use. *N Engl J Med.* 2001;345:351–358. 3) Hollander JE, et al. Management of Cocaine Associated Myocardial Ischemia. *N Engl J Med.* 1995;333:1267–1272.

VALVULAR DISEASE

Does my patient with aortic stenosis need surgery?

KEY CONCEPT	The decision to refer a patient with aortic stenosis (AS) for surgery is based on the presence of symptoms, severity of AS, left ventricular function, and whether they require other surgeries involving the heart.
HISTORY	HPI: Dyspnea with exertion, angina, syncope, or orthopnea. Sometimes patients adjust there lifestyle subconsciously to avoid exertion. PMH: Hypertension, coronary artery disease, rheumatic fever/heart disease, hyperlipidemia. PSH: Valve replacement, prior thoracotomy. FH: Congenital bicuspid aortic valve.
PHYSICAL EXAM	Mid-late peaking systolic ejection murmur with radiation to carotids, paradoxically split S2, diminished carotid upstroke, evidence of heart failure (elevated JVP, rales, S3, peripheral edema).
ELECTRO-CARDIOGRAM	Left ventricular hypertrophy with strain pattern, left axis deviation.
IMAGING	**Echo:** Assess aortic valve area, pressure across the aortic valve, morphology (ex. Calcified or bicuspid). Assess left ventricle size and function.
SYNTHESIS	**SYM** = **SYM**ptomatic (See HPI). **ASYM** = **ASYM**ptomatic. **CARD-SUR** = Patient is due for **CARD**iac **SUR**gery for reasons other than the aortic stenosis (ex. CABG). **MOD-AS** = **MOD**erate **A**ortic **S**tenosis by echocardiography. **SEV-AS** = **SEV**ere **A**ortic **S**tenosis by echocardiography. **LVSD** = **L**eft **V**entricular **S**ystolic **D**ysfunction with ejection fraction < 0.50. **FOLLOW** = Clinical **FOLLOW** up and annual echocardiogram or sooner if symptoms develop. If a patient has severe aortic stenosis very close follow up is needed and consideration should be given for exercise stress testing to objectively determine if a patient is genuinely asymptomatic. **LG-AS** = **L**ow **G**radient **A**ortic **S**tenosis. If LV function is low it is possible the LV cannot generate enough pressure to reveal the true severe gradient across the aortic valve. Consider dobutamine echo to enhance LV function. If LV function improves significantly and severe aortic stenosis is seen, refer for AVR. **AVR** = Refer for **A**ortic **V**alve **R**eplacement. If patient is due for cardiac surgery for other reasons, AVR is performed at the same time to reduce perioperative risk and need for repeat thoracotomy.

EPIPHANY	MOD-AS + ASYM = FOLLOW MOD-AS + ASYM + CARD-SUR = AVR MOD-AS + SYM = AVR MOD-AS + LVSD = LG-AS SEV-AS + ASYM = FOLLOW SEV-AS + ASYM + CARD-SUR = AVR SEV-AS + ASYM + LVSD = AVR SEV-AS + SYM = AVR
DISCUSSION	In patients with severe symptomatic aortic stenosis the survival rate is 2 to 3 years unless AVR is performed.
CONTRA-INDICATIONS	– The most common cause of death in asymptomatic valve disease is surgery! Use careful consideration in determining if symptoms are genuinely present and in deciding when to time surgery.
PEARLS	– 1.0–2.0% of the population born with a bicuspid aortic valve. – AVR is less beneficial in patients where low ejection fraction is caused by depressed contractility compared to increased afterload. Left ventricular function may be evaluated with a dobutamine echocardiogram, which will also rule out possibility of pseudo aortic stenosis. – Mild aortic regurgitation present in 80% of patients with AS.
REFERENCE	1) Bonow RO, et al. ACC/AHA Guidelines for the Management of Patients with Valvular Heart Disease. *J Am Coll Cardiol.* 2006;48:e1–e148. 2) Carabello BA. Clinical practice: aortic stenosis. *N Engl J Med.* 2002;346:677–682.

Does my patient with aortic regurgitation need surgery?

KEY CONCEPT	The decision to refer a patient with aortic regurgitation (AR) for surgery is based on symptoms, severity of AR, left ventricular function, and whether they require other surgeries involving the heart.
HISTORY	HPI: Dyspnea with exertion, angina, syncope, or orthopnea. PMH: Aortic dissection, bacterial endocarditis, hypertension, rheumatic heart disease.
PHYSICAL EXAM	Corrigan pulse, decrescendo diastolic murmur, mid-diastolic apical rumble (Austin Flint murmur).
ELECTRO-CARDIOGRAM	Left ventricular hypertrophy.
IMAGING	**Echo:** Assess aortic valve structure, any evidence of concomitant stenosis, grade severity of regurgitation. Assess left ventricle size and function.
SYNTHESIS	**SYM** = **SYM**ptomatic (See HPI). **ASYM** = **ASYM**ptomatic. **CARD-SUR** = Patient is due for **CARD**iac **SUR**gery for reasons other than the aortic regurgitation (ex. CABG). **MOD-AR** = **MOD**erate **A**ortic **R**egurgitation by echocardiography. **SEV-AR** = **SEV**ere **A**ortic **R**egurgitation by echocardiography. **LVSD** = **L**eft **V**entricular **S**ystolic **D**ysfunction with ejection fraction < 0.50. **INFXN** = Infection: Severe aortic regurgitation resulting from infective endocarditis. This can be particularly devastating when the aortic regurgitation is acute. Infections often will not be successfully treated medically and resolution of the infection will not restore competency to the valve. **FOLLOW** = Clinical **FOLLOW** up and annual echocardiogram or sooner if symptoms develop. If a patient has severe aortic regurgitation very close follow up is needed and consideration should be given for exercise stress testing to objectively determine if a patient is genuinely asymptomatic. **AVR** = Refer for **A**ortic **V**alve **R**eplacement. If patient due for cardiac surgery for other reasons, AVR is performed at the same time to reduce perioperative risk and need for repeat thoracotomy.

E EPIPHANY	**MOD-AR + ASYM = FOLLOW** **MOD-AR + ASYM + CARD-SUR = AVR** **MOD-AR + SYM = AVR** **SEV-AR + ASYM = FOLLOW** **SEV-AR + ASYM + CARD-SUR = AVR** **SEV-AR + ASYM + LVSD = AVR** **SEV-AR + INFXN = AVR** **SEV-AR + SYM = AVR**
DISCUSSION	Patients with severe aortic regurgitation determined by echocardiogram should be referred for aortic valve replacement if they are symptomatic or have evidence of structural remodeling that will lead to heart failure.
CONTRA-INDICATIONS	– The most common cause of death in asymptomatic valve disease is surgery! Use careful consideration in determining if symptoms are genuinely present and in deciding when to time surgery.
PEARLS	– AVR is associated with a mortality rate of 4% when performed in isolation and 7% when performed with CABG. – Outcomes for AVR are better in patients with a left ventricular end-systolic dimension <55 mm and a left ventricular ejection fraction >55%.
REFERENCE	1) Bonow RO, et al. ACC/AHA Guidelines for the Management of Patients with Valvular Heart Disease. *J Am Coll Cardiol.* 2006;48:e1–e148. 2) Enriquez-Sarano M, et al. Clinical practice. Aortic regurgitation. *N Engl J Med.* 2004;351:1539–1546. 3) Bekeredjian R, et al. Valvular Heart Disease: Aortic Regurgitation. *Circulation.* 2005;112:125–134.

Does my patient with mitral stenosis need surgery?

KEY CONCEPT	The decision to refer a patient with mitral stenosis for surgery or percutaneous intervention is based on valve morphology, degree of stenosis, symptoms, left atrial thrombus, and concomitant mitral regurgitation.
HISTORY	HPI: Dyspnea on exertion, chest pain, atrial fibrillation, or thromboembolic event. PMH: Rheumatic heart disease.
PHYSICAL EXAM	Opening snap, accentuated S1, low-pitched mid-diastolic rumble, right ventricular heave, diminished apical impulse.
ELECTRO-CARDIOGRAM	Left atrial enlargement, right ventricular hypertrophy, or atrial fibrillation.
IMAGING	ECHO: Doming of anterior mitral valve (MV) leaflet, "hockey stick" appearance of anterior MV leaflet, immobility of posterior MV leaflet, MV annular calcification, thickening of MV leaflet. X-ray: Left atrial enlargement, calcification of MV annulus, enlargement of pulmonary artery.
SYNTHESIS	**MS-ECHO** = Moderate (mean gradient 5–10 mm Hg, pulmonary artery systolic pressure (PASP) 30–50 mm Hg, valve area 1–1.5 cm^2) or severe (mean gradient >10 mm Hg, PASP >10 mm Hg, valve area <1 cm^2) **M**itral **S**tenosis on **ECHO**cardiogram. **PCMBV** = Refer patient for **P**er**C**utaneous **M**itral **V**alve **B**alloon **V**alvotomy. **FVM** = **F**avorable Mitral **V**alve **M**orphology for PCMBV. **UFVM** = **U**n**F**avorable Mitral **V**alve **M**orphology for PCMBV. **MVR** = Refer patient for **M**itral **V**alve **R**epair/Replacement. **LATH** = **L**eft **A**trial **TH**rombus. **MSMR** = **M**oderate or **S**evere **M**itral **R**egurgitation. **SYMP** = **SYMP**toms of dyspnea on exertion or at rest. Limitation in performing ordinary activities. **PHTN** = Pulmonary hypertension (pulmonary artery systolic pressure >50 mm Hg). **ASYM** = No symptoms on presentation or concomitant conditions. **MED** = Yearly evaluation with history, physical exam, chest X-ray, and electrocardiogram. Yearly echocardiogram in severe mitral stenosis or patient with change in clinical.

 EPIPHANY	**MS-ECHO + FVM + SYMP = PCMBV** **MS-ECHO + FVM + PHTN = PCMBV** **MS-ECHO + UFVM = MVR** **MS-ECHO + LATH = MVR** **MS-ECHO + MSMR = MVR** **MS-ECHO + ASYM = MED**
 DISCUSSION	Percutaneous balloon mitral valve valvotomy is the preferred intervention in patients with moderate to severe mitral stenosis with favorable valve morphology who are symptomatic or have pulmonary hypertension.
 CONTRA-INDICATIONS	– PCMBV should not be performed in patients with moderate to severe mitral regurgitation (make symptoms worse) or presence of a left atrial thrombus (may embolize and form thrombus systemically).
 PEARLS	– In the presence of significant calcification, fibrosis, and subvalvular fusion of the MV leaflets, PCMBV is less likely to be successful, and MVR is the preferred intervention.
 REFERENCE	1) Bonow RO, et al. ACC/AHA 2008 Update of Valvular Heart Disease. *J Am Coll Cardiol.* 2006;48:e1–e148. 2) Carabello BA. Modern Management of Mitral Stenosis. *Circulation.* 2005;112:432–437.

Does my patient with mitral regurgitation need surgery?

KEY CONCEPT	The decision of surgical intervention in a patient with mitral regurgitation is based upon symptomatology and degree of left ventricular (LV) dysfunction.
HISTORY	HPI: Symptoms of dyspnea, exercise intolerance, or fatigue. PMH: Mitral valve prolapse, coronary artery disease, rheumatic heart disease, collagen vascular disease.
PHYSICAL EXAM	Apical holosystolic murmur radiating to axilla, displaced apical impulse.
ELECTRO-CARDIOGRAM	Left atrial (LA) and LV enlargement.
IMAGING	ECHO: LA and LV enlargement; LV ejection fraction <0.6. Calcification of mitral annulus or leaflet. X-ray: LA and LV enlargement, pulmonary edema, increased pulmonary vascularity.
SYNTHESIS	**SMR-ECHO** = **S**evere **M**itral **R**egurgitation on **ECHO**: dilated LA and LV; regurgitant volume >=60 mL/beat, regurgitant fraction >=50%, regurgitant orifice >=40 cm², abnormal flail leaflets. **MVR** = Refer for **M**itral **V**alve **R**epair/**R**eplacement. **MED** = Continue with patients' medical therapy and follow up with echocardiogram yearly or sooner if symptoms develop. **ASYM** = No symptoms on presentation. **SYMP** = **SYMP**toms of dyspnea, exercise intolerance, or fatigue. **LVSD** = Left ventricular ejection fraction <0.60. **ESD** = **E**nd **S**ystolic **D**imension >=40 mm. **AFIB** = New-onset **A**trial **FIB**rillation (**AFIB**) **PHTN** = **P**ulmonary **H**yper**T**ensio**N**: pulmonary artery systolic pressure >50 mm Hg at rest or >60 mm Hg at exercise.
E **EPIPHANY**	**SMR-ECHO + SYMP = MVR** **SMR-ECHO + LVSD = MVR** **SMR-ECHO + ESD = MVR** **SMR-ECHO + AFIB = MVR** **SMR-ECHO + PHTN = MVR** **SMR-ECHO + ASYM = MED**
DISCUSSION	Patients with severe mitral regurgitation determined by echocardiogram should be referred for mitral valve replacement or repair if they are symptomatic, have evidence of left ventricular dilation or dysfunction, have pulmonary hypertension, or develop atrial fibrillation.

 CONTRA- INDICATIONS	– Mitral valve surgery is not indicated for asymptomatic patients with mitral regurgitation and preserved LV function, where significant doubt of feasibility of repair exists.
 PEARLS	– Mitral valve repair when compared to mitral valve replacement has been shown to have a lower operative mortality rate and better longer-term survival and so is preferred if feasible.
REFERENCE	1) Bonow RO, et al. Guideline Update of Valvular Heart Disease. *J Am Coll Cardiol.* 2006;48:e1–e148. 2) Foster E. Mitral Regurgitation Due to Regenerative Mitral Valve Disease. *N Engl J Med.* 2010;363:156–165. 3) Carabello BA. The Current Therapy for Mitral Regurgitation. *J Am Coll Cardiol.* 2008;52:319–326.

How do I manage my pregnant patient with mitral stenosis?

KEY CONCEPT	The management of pregnant patients with mitral stenosis (MS) is based upon the presence of symptoms, mitral valve morphologic features. Treatment of a pregnant woman with MS is limited to those who are symptomatic.
HISTORY	HPI: Dyspnea on exertion, chest pain, atrial fibrillation, or thromboembolic event. PMH: Rheumatic heart disease.
PHYSICAL EXAM	Opening snap, accentuated S1, low-pitched mid-diastolic rumble, right ventricular heave, diminished apical impulse.
ELECTRO-CARDIOGRAM	Left atrial enlargement, right ventricular hypertrophy, or atrial fibrillation.
IMAGING	ECHO: Doming of anterior mitral valve (MV) leaflet, "hockey stick" appearance of anterior MV leaflet, immobility of posterior MV leaflet, MV annular calcification, thickening of MV leaflet. X-ray: Left atrial enlargement, calcification of mitral valve annulus, enlargement of pulmonary artery.
SYNTHESIS	**PREG-MS** = **PREG**nant patient with documented **M**itral **S**tenosis. **SYMP** = **SYMP**toms of dyspnea on exertion or at rest, limitation in performing ordinary activities, orthopnea, or pulmonary edema unresponsive to medical treatment. **ASYM** = Patient is **ASYM**ptomatic. **MED** = **MED**ical treatment with furosemide 80 mg/day and metoprolol 25 mg/day. **PCBMV** = Refer patient for **P**er**C**utaneous **B**alloon **M**itral **V**alvuloplasty. **SURG** = Refer patient for **SURG**ery with either mitral valve repair or replacement. **UFM** = **U**n**F**avorable **M**itral valve morphology for PCMBV.
E EPIPHANY	**PREG-MS + ASYM = MED** **PREG-MS + SYMP = PCBMV** **PREG-MS + SYMP + UFM = SURG**
DISCUSSION	Patients with severe MS who are symptomatic prior to conception will not tolerate the hemodynamic burden of pregnancy and should be considered for PCBMV if valve morphology is favorable prior to conception.

CONTRA-INDICATIONS	– PCMBV should not be performed in patients with moderate to severe mitral regurgitation or presence of a left atrial thrombus.
PEARLS	– Pregnant women with mitral stenosis develop symptoms most commonly in the 2nd and 3rd trimesters. – In patients with a favorable valve morphology PCMBV has been associated with a lower rate in fetal and neonatal mortality compared to mitral valve repair or replacement.
REFERENCE	1) Bonow RO, et al. 2008 ACC/AHA Guideline Update on Valvular Heart Disease. *J Am Coll Cardiol*. 2006;48:e1–e148.

Does my patient with tricuspid regurgitation need surgery?

KEY CONCEPT	The decision to refer a patient with tricuspid regurgitation (TR) for surgery is based upon symptoms and coexisting tricuspid valve morphology.
HISTORY	HPI: Patient presenting with palpitations, edema, and SOB. PMH: Rheumatic heart disease, infective endocarditis, Marfan's syndrome, Ebstein's anomaly (funnel-shaped tricuspid valve). PSH: Endomyocardial biopsy, radiation therapy.
PHYSICAL EXAM	Holosystolic murmur best heard at the right mid-sternal border, right ventricular heave (present on palpation of left sternal border), jugular venous distension, ascites, hepatomegaly.
ELECTRO-CARDIOGRAM	Nonspecific ST-T wave changes.
IMAGING	ECHO: Dilated right atrium and right ventricle, dilated tricuspid annulus, vena contracta width >0.7 cm and systolic flow reversal in hepatic veins. X-ray: Right atrial enlargement, prominent azygous vein, pleural effusion.
SYNTHESIS	**S-TR** = **S**evere **T**ricuspid **R**egurgitation (vena contracta width >0.7 cm and systolic flow reversal in hepatic veins). **MVD** = **M**itral **V**alve **D**isease requiring surgery. **SYMP** = Patient with **SYMP**toms of dyspnea, palpitations, fatigue, or weakness. **AB-TVL** = **AB**normal **T**ricuspid **V**alve **L**eaflets not amenable to annuloplasty or repair. **MED** = **MED**ical management with yearly echocardiogram or sooner if development of symptoms. **SURG-T** = Refer patient for **SURG**ical repair or replacement of **T**ricuspid valve.
EPIPHANY	**S-TR = MED** **S-TR + SYMP = SURG-T** **S-TR + MVD = SURG-T** **S-TR + AB-TVL = SURG-T**
DISCUSSION	In patients with tricuspid valve leaflet morphology where repair is feasible, it is preferred because of ease of operation and faster recovery period; however, repair is associated with a higher rate of recurrent TR.

 CONTRA-INDICATIONS	Tricuspid valve replacement or annuloplasty is not indicated in asymptomatic patients with TR whose pulmonary artery systolic pressure is less than 60 mm Hg in the presence of a normal MV.
 PEARLS	– Operative mortality rates for patients with TR undergoing tricuspid valve repair with concomitant surgery on another valve ranged from 6–14%. – In patients with symptomatic TR, surgery should be performed before the development of a right ventricular end-systolic area $>=20$ cm^2 or anemia with hemoglobin $<=11.3$ g/dL as it is associated with a higher rate of event-free survival.
 REFERENCE	1) Bonow RO, et al. ACC/AHA 2008 Guideline Update on Valvular Heart Disease: Focused Update on Infective Endocarditis. *J Am Coll Cardiol.* 2006;48:e1–e148.

Does my patient have endocarditis?

 KEY CONCEPT	The diagnosis of endocarditis is based upon the presence of major and minor Duke's criteria.
 HISTORY	HPI: Symptoms of fever and/or new-onset murmur. PMH: Congenital heart disease, prior infective endocarditis, mitral valve prolapse. PSH: Mechanical heart valve. SH: IV drug use.
 PHYSICAL EXAM	New-onset valvular regurgitation murmur, splinter hemorrhage, conjunctival petechiae, Janeway lesion, Osler node, Roth spots.
 IMAGING	ECHO: Echogenic oscillating intracardiac mass, periannular abscess, dehiscence of MHV.
SYNTHESIS	**Duke's Criteria** **MAJOR = MAJOR** criteria are: (1) two separate positive blood culture for infective endocarditis (*Staphylococcus aureus, Viridans streptococci*, HACEK, or *Streptococcus bovis*); (2) endocardial involvement (echocardiogram or new valvular regurgitation murmur). **MINOR = MINOR** criteria are: (1) fever; (2) predisposition (IV drug use, cardiac condition); (3) vascular phenomena (arterial embolism, Janeway lesion, conjunctival hemorrhage, or septic pulmonary embolus); (4) immunologic phenomena (Roth spots, Osler nodes, glomerulonephritis, or rheumatoid factor); (5) microbiologic evidence (positive blood culture not meeting major criterion). **1MAJOR** = Patient has 1 major Duke criteria. **2MAJOR** = Patient has both major Duke criteria. **3MINOR** = Patient has 3 or 4 minor Duke criteria. **5MINOR** = Patient has 5 minor Duke criteria. **EC** = Patient has **E**ndo**C**arditis based on Duke's criteria.
 EPIPHANY	**2MAJOR = EC** **1MAJOR + 3MINOR = EC** **5MINOR = EC**

DISCUSSION	Duke's criteria are a collection of major and minor criteria based upon findings on physical exam, imaging, and microbiologic findings. A patient with 2 major, 1 major and 3 minor, or 5 minor criteria is diagnostic for endocarditis.
PEARLS	– TTE and TEE may produce false-negative results if vegetations are small or have already embolized. – *Staphylococcus aureus* is the most common cause of infective endocarditis.
REFERENCE	1) Baddour LM, et al. Infective Endocarditis. *Circulation*. 2005;111: e394–e434. 2) Mylonakis E, et al. Infective Endocarditis in Adults. *N Engl J Med*. 2001; 345:1318–1330.

Does my patient need endocarditis prophylaxis?

KEY CONCEPT	The decision to begin infective endocarditis (IE) prophylaxis is based upon the presence of cardiac abnormalities/risk factors and the type of procedure performed.
HISTORY	HPI: Patient with underlying cardiac condition undergoing surgery or invasive procedure. PMH: IE, congenital heart disease (CHD), mechanical heart valve (MHV), mitral valve prolapse, rheumatic heart disease. PSH: Valve replacement, CHD defect repair, cardiac transplant.
PHYSICAL EXAM	Murmur, sternotomy scar.
IMAGING	ECHO: MHV, CHD, severe native valvular heart disease.
SYNTHESIS	**HIGHR** = Patient with any one of the following cardiac conditions are considered at **HIGH R**isk for adverse outcomes from IE: MHV; previous IE; unrepaired CHD, including palliative stents and conduits; completely repaired CHD with prosthetic material or device during first 6 months following procedure; repaired CHD with residual defects at the site or adjacent to the site of a prosthetic patch or prosthetic device; cardiac transplant recipients who develop cardiac valvulopathy. **DP** = **D**ental **P**rocedures involving manipulation of gingival tissue or perforation of oral mucosa. **GI/GU** = **G**astro**I**ntestinal or **G**enito**U**rinary tract procedures including endoscopy, colonoscopy, cystoscopy, vaginal delivery, and hysterectomy. **RSP** = **R**e**SP**iratory tract procedure involving incision of respiratory tract (biopsy, drainage of abscess, or empyema). **ISMS** = surgery involving **I**nfected **S**kin, skin stricture, or **M**usculo**S**keletal tissue. **DPR** = Prophylaxis for DP is amoxicillin 2 g oral or ampicillin 2 g IV if unable to tolerate oral. If allergic to penicillin give clindamycin 600 mg oral or if unable to tolerate oral give IV. **RPR** = Prophylaxis for RSP is amoxicillin 2 g oral or ampicillin 2 g IV if unable to tolerate oral. If allergic to penicillin, give vancomycin 1 g oral or if unable to tolerate give IV. **IPR** = Prophylaxis for ISM is amoxicillin 2 g oral or ampicillin 2 g IV if unable to tolerate oral. If allergic to penicillin, give clindamycin 600 mg oral or if unable to tolerate oral give IV. **NP** = **N**o **P**rophylaxis.

 EPIPHANY	**HIGHR + DP = DPR** **HIGHR + RSP = RPR** **HIGHR + ISMS = IPR** **HIGHR + GI/GU = NP**
 DISCUSSION	IE prophylaxis is recommended in patients with cardiac conditions that are considered high risk for outcomes from IE undergoing DP, RSP, or ISM procedures. Prophylaxis is not recommended in GI/GU procedures.
 PEARLS	– If the dosage of antibiotic is inadvertently not administered before the procedure, the dosage may be administered up to 2 hours after the procedure. – Overall mortality rate for both native and prosthetic-valve endocarditis remains as high as 20–25% with death resulting from CNS embolic events and hemodynamic compromise.
 REFERENCE	1) Wilson W, et al. Prevention of Infective Endocarditis: Guidelines from the American Heart Association. *Circulation.* 2007;116:1736–1754. 2) Mylonakis E, et al. Infective Endocarditis in Adults. *N Engl J Med.* 2001;345:1318–1330.

Should I refer my patient with native valve endocarditis for surgery?

KEY CONCEPT	The decision to refer a patient with native valve endocarditis (NVE) for surgery is based upon the presence of complications.
HISTORY	HPI: Dyspnea on exertion, fatigue, weakness. PMH: Congenital heart disease, prior infective endocarditis, mitral valve prolapse. PSH: Intravenous drug use.
PHYSICAL EXAM	Decrescendo diastolic murmur, mid-diastolic apical rumble (Austin Flint murmur); apical holosystolic murmur radiating to axilla, displaced apical impulse; splinter hemorrhage, conjunctival petechiae, Janeway lesion (erythematous nodular lesion on palms or soles), Roth spots (retinal hemorrhage with pale center), Osler node (painful red raised lesion on hands or feet).
IMAGING	ECHO = Echogenic oscillating intracardiac mass, periannular abscess, left atrial and ventricular enlargement, left ventricular ejection fraction <40%, wall motion abnormalities.
SYNTHESIS	**NVE** = Patient diagnosed with **N**ative **V**alve **E**ndocarditis. **SURG** = Refer patient for **SURG**ical treatment with valve repair or replacement. **HF** = Patient with **H**eart **F**ailure (dyspnea on exertion or at rest, fatigue, weakness). **S-REG** = Patient with **S**evere aortic or mitral **REG**urgitation with hemodynamic abnormalities such as elevated left ventricular end-diastolic pressure or premature closure of mitral valve with aortic regurgitation. **UMT-F** = Endocarditis **U**nresponsive to **M**edical **T**reatment or due to fungal infections. **COMP** = Cardiovascular **COMP**lications of endocarditis: heart block, perivalvular abscess, or fistula formation.
EPIPHANY	**NVE + HF = SURG** **NVE + S-REG = SURG** **NVE + UMT-F = SURG** **NVE + COMP = SURG**

DISCUSSION	In patients with NVE where surgery is indicated, valve repair is preferred over replacement as it is associated with lower operative mortality and long-term outcome.
PEARLS	– Patients with a history of intravenous drug use and human immunodeficiency virus are at increased risk for recurrent infection and reoperation.
REFERENCE	1) Bonow RO, et al. 2008 Guideline Update of Valvular Heart Disease. *J Am Coll Cardiol.* 2006;48:e1. 2) Fedoruk LM, et al. Predictors of Recurrence and Reoperation for Prosthetic Valve Endocarditis after Valve Replacement Surgery for Native Valve Endocarditis. *Thorac Cardiovasc Surg.* 2009;137:326–333.

How do I medically treat prosthetic valve endocarditis?

KEY CONCEPT	The choice of antibiotics administered in a patient with prosthetic valve infective endocarditis is based upon blood culture results and allergies to beta-lactam antibiotics.
HISTORY	HPI: Symptoms of fever and/or new-onset murmur. PMH: Congenital heart disease, prior infective endocarditis, mitral valve prolapse. PSH: Heart valve replacement. SH: IV drug use.
PHYSICAL EXAM	New-onset valvular regurgitation murmur, splinter hemorrhage, conjunctival petechiae, Janeway lesion (erythematous nodular lesion on palms or soles), Roth spots (retinal hemorrhage with pale center), Osler node (painful red raised lesion on hands or feet).
IMAGING	ECHO: Echogenic oscillating intracardiac mass, periannular abscess, dehiscence of mechanical heart valve.
SYNTHESIS	**PVIE** = Patient with **P**rosthetic **V**alve **I**nfective **E**ndocarditis. **STREP** = 2 positive blood cultures for *Viridans* **STREP**tococci or *Streptococcus bovis*. **STAPH** = 2 positive blood cultures for ***STAPH**ylococcus aureus*. **ENTRC** = 2 positive blood cultures for **ENT**e**R**ococci. **HACEK** = 2 positive blood cultures for HACEK organisms (***H**aemophilus aphrophilus*, ***A**ctinobacillus actinomycetemcomitans*, ***C**ardiobacterium hominis*, ***E**ikenella corrodens*, or ***K**ingella kingae*). **CNEG** = **C**ulture **NEG**ative endocarditis (endocarditis without etiology following inoculation of 3 blood samples in a standard blood culture system). **ABL** = Patient **A**llergic to **B**eta-**L**actam antibiotics. **CTX-6** = Ceftriaxone 2 g/24 hr IV for 6 weeks. **CTX-4** = Ceftriaxone 2 g/24 hr IV for 4 weeks. **GENT-2** = **GENT**amycin 3 mg/kg per 24 hours IV in 3 equally divided doses for 2 weeks. **GENT-6** = **GENT**amycin 3 mg/kg per 24 hours IV in 3 equally divided doses for 6 weeks. **NAF** = **NAF**cillin 12 g/24 hr IV in 6 equally divided doses for 6 weeks. **RIF** = **RIF**ampin 900 mg/24 hr IV in 3 equally divided doses for 6 weeks. **AMP** = **AMP**icillin-sulbactam 12 grams per 24 hours IV in 4 equally divided doses for 4 weeks. **VANC** = **VANC**omycin 30 mg/kg per 24 hours IV in 2 equally divided doses for 6 weeks. **CIPRO** = **CIPRO**floxacin 800 mg/24 hours IV in 2 equally divided doses for 4 weeks.

EPIPHANY	**PVIE + STREP = CTX-6 + GECT** **PVIE + STAPH = NAF + RIF + GENT** **PVIE + ENTRC = AMP** **PVIE + HACEK = CTX-4** **PVIE + STREP + ABL = VANC** **PVIE + STREP + ABL = VANC + RIF + GENT** **PVIE + ENTRC + ABL = VANC + GENT-6** **PVIE + HACEK + ABL = CIPRO**
DISCUSSION	Patients with prosthetic valve endocarditis should be administered with the appropriate antibiotics based upon sensitivity and blood culture findings.
PEARLS	– Endocarditis caused by *Staphylococcus aureus* is associated with a lower mortality rate than streptococcal infection. – The risk of embolization is decreased after the institution of effective antimicrobial therapy in patients with infective endocarditis.
REFERENCE	1) Baddour LM, et al. Infective endocarditis: diagnosis, antimicrobial therapy, and management of complications: a statement for healthcare professionals from the Committee on Rheumatic Fever, Endocarditis, and Kawasaki Disease, Council on Cardiovascular Disease in the Young, and the Councils on Clinical Cardiology, Stroke, and Cardiovascular Surgery and Anesthesia, American Heart Association: endorsed by the Infectious Diseases Society of America. *Circulation*. 2005;111:e394–e434.

Should I refer my patient with prosthetic valve endocarditis for surgery?

KEY CONCEPT	The decision to refer a patient with prosthetic valve endocarditis (PVE) for surgery is based upon the presence of complications.
HISTORY	HPI: Dyspnea on exertion, fatigue, weakness. PMH: Congenital heart disease, prior infective endocarditis, mitral valve prolapse. PSH: Prosthetic valve replacement. SH: Intravenous drug use.
PHYSICAL EXAM	Decrescendo diastolic murmur, mid-diastolic apical rumble (Austin Flint murmur); apical holosystolic murmur radiating to axilla, displaced apical impulse; splinter hemorrhage, conjunctival petechiae, Janeway lesion (erythematous nodular lesion on palms or soles), Roth spots (retinal hemorrhage with pale center), Osler node (painful red raised lesion on hands or feet).
IMAGING	ECHO: Echogenic oscillating intracardiac mass, periannular abscess, left atrial and ventricular enlargement, left ventricular ejection fraction <40%, wall motion abnormalities.
SYNTHESIS	**PVE** = Patient diagnosed with **P**rosthetic **V**alve **E**ndocarditis. **SURG** = Refer patient for **SURG**ical treatment with valve repair or replacement. **HF** = Patient with **H**eart **F**ailure (dyspnea on exertion or at rest, fatigue, weakness). **REG** = Patient with increasing valve obstruction or worsening **REG**urgitation. **UMT-F** = Endocarditis **U**nresponsive to **M**edical **T**reatment or due to **F**ungal infections. **COMP** = **COMP**lications of endocarditis such as heart block, perivalvular abscess, or fistula formation.
EPIPHANY	**PVE + HF = SURG** **PVE + REG = SURG** **PVE + UMT-F = SURG** **PVE + COMP = SURG**

 DISCUSSION	In patients with PVE where surgery is indicated, valve repair is preferred over replacement as it is associated with lower operative mortality and long-term outcome.
 PEARLS	– Patients with a history of intravenous drug use and human immunodeficiency virus are at increased risk for recurrent infection and reoperation. – Long-term mortality is increased in patients who develop PVE within 6 months of surgery.
 REFERENCE	1) Bonow RO, et al. ACC/AHA 2008 Guideline Update on Valvular Heart Disease: Focused Update on Infective Endocarditis. *J Am Coll Cardiol.* 2008;118:887–896.

How do I medically treat endocarditis?

KEY CONCEPT	The choice of antibiotics administered in a patient with native valve infective endocarditis is based upon blood culture results.
HISTORY	HPI: Symptoms of fever and/or new onset murmur. PMH: Congenital heart disease, prior infective endocarditis, mitral valve prolapse. PSH: Mechanical heart valve. SH: IV drug use.
PHYSICAL EXAM	New-onset valvular regurgitation murmur, splinter hemorrhage, conjunctival petechiae, Janeway lesion, Osler node, Roth spots.
IMAGING	ECHO: Echogenic oscillating intracardiac mass, periannular abscess, dehiscence of MHV.
SYNTHESIS	**NVIE** = Patient with **N**ative **V**alve **I**nfective **E**ndocarditis. **STREP** = 2 positive blood cultures for *Viridans* streptococci or *Streptococcus bovis*. **STAPH** = 2 positive blood cultures for *Staphylococcus aureus*. **ENTR** = 2 positive blood cultures for enterococci. **HACEK** = 2 positive blood cultures for HACEK organisms (***H**aemophilus aphrophilus*, ***A**ctinobacillus actinomycetemcomitans*, ***C**ardiobacterium hominis*, ***E**ikenella corrodens*, or ***K**ingella kingae*). **CXNEG** = Culture negative endocarditis (endocarditis without etiology following inoculation of 3 blood samples in a standard blood culture system). **CTX-GENT** = Ceftriaxone 2 g/24 hr IV and Gentamycin 3 mg/kg per 24 hours IV for 2 weeks. **NAF-GENT** = Nafcillin 12 g/24hr IV in 6 equally divided doses for 6 weeks and Gentamycin 3 mg/kg per 24 hours IV in 3 equally divided doses for 3 days. **AS-GENT** = Ampicillin-sulbactam 12 grams per 24 hours IV in 4 equally divided doses for 4 weeks and Gentamycin 3 mg/kg per 24 hours IV in 3 equally divided doses for 4 weeks. **AMP** = Ampicillin 12 g/24 hr IV in 6 equally divided doses, for 4 weeks. **CEF** = Ceftriaxone 2 g/24 hr IV for 4 weeks.
EPIPHANY	**NVIE + STREP = CTX-GENT** **NVIE + STAPH = NAF-GENT** **NVIE + ENTRC = AMP** **NVIE + HACEK = CEF** **NVIE + CXNEG = AS-GENT**

DISCUSSION	Patients with native valve endocarditis should be administered with the appropriate antibiotics based upon sensitivity and blood culture findings.
CONTRA-INDICATIONS	– For patients with IE and **STREP** who cannot tolerate beta-lactam antibiotics, give vancomycin 30 mg/kg per 24 hours IV in 2 equally divided doses for 4 weeks. – For patients with IE and **STAPH** who cannot tolerate beta-lactam antibiotics, give vancomycin 30 mg/kg per 24 hours IV in 2 equally divided doses for 6 weeks. – For patients with IE and **ENTRC** who cannot tolerate beta-lactam antibiotics, give vancomycin 30 mg/kg per 24 hours IV in 2 equally divided doses and gentamycin 3 mg/kg per 24 hours IV in 3 equally divided doses for 6 weeks. – For patients with IE and **HACEK** who cannot tolerate beta-lactam antibiotics, give ciprofloxacin 800 mg/24 hours IV in 2 equally divided doses. – For patients with IE and **CXNEG**, give ciprofloxacin 800 mg/24 hours IV in 2 equally divided doses.
PEARLS	– Endocarditis caused *Staphylococcus aureus* is associated with a lower mortality rate than streptococcal infection. – The risk of embolization is decreased after the institution of effective antimicrobial therapy in patients with infective endocarditis.
REFERENCE	1) Baddour LM. Infective Endocarditis: Diagnosis, Antimicrobial Therapy, and Management Complications *Circulation*. 2005;111:e394–e434.

How to manage an infected pacemaker?

KEY CONCEPT	A cardiac device infection is confirmed on positive cultures from the generator pocket, lead, or blood (in the presence of local inflammatory signs at generator pocket or absence of another source of bacteremia and resolution of blood stream infection after device explantation). Pocket infections involve the subcutaneous pocket containing the device and the subcutaneous segment of the leads. Deeper infections involve the transvenous portion of the lead with associated bacteremia and/or endovascular infection.
HISTORY	Recent manipulation of the device, particularly elective secondary manipulations such as generator exchange, newly implanted device, device revision, or generator change. Temporary pacing prior to permanent device placement.
PHYSICAL EXAM	Systemic symptoms: Fever, chills, malaise, anorexia, nausea, sweating symptomatic heart failure. Pacemaker site: Pocket infection: local signs of inflammation at the generator pocket, including swelling, erythema, warmth, tenderness, drainage, purulent drainage, skin ulceration, and generator/lead erosion
IMAGING	TEE-vegetations can occur anywhere along the course of the electrode, including the endocardium of the right atrium or right ventricle. CXR for pneumonia, empyema, lung abscess.
SYNTHESIS (cont. on next page)	**INPM** = **IN**fected **Pa**ce**M**aker. **PPBC** = **P**ersistent **P**ositive **B**lood **C**ulture (patients with persistently positive blood cultures should be treated for at least 4 weeks with antimicrobials even if TEE is negative for vegetations or other evidence of infection). **T4W** = **T**reatment for at least **4 W**eeks. **DR** = **D**evice **R**emoval (device and leads removed, regardless of clinical presentation). **Indications for device removal:** 1) If there is clinical or echocardiographic evidence of pacemaker/AICD infection. 2) If there is no other source identified for SAB. 3) If there is relapsing SAB after a course of appropriate antibiotic therapy. **AMT** = **A**ntimicrobial **T**herapy. **GS-BCX** = Gram stain and culture and lead tip culture should be obtained. All patients should have at least two sets of blood cultures drawn at initial evaluation. Document negative cultures. Blood cultures should be repeated in all patients after device removal. **PNI** = **P**acemaker **N**ot **I**nfected.

 SYNTHESIS (cont. from previous page)	**SD** = **S**alvage **D**evice: patients with bacteremia from a defined source other than the device (including valvular infection) if the following conditions are met: no clinical/TEE evidence of lead infection; no evidence of pocket infection; and device has not been manipulated. Treated with antibiotics for the bacteremic disease and then observed for relapse. Subsequent unexplained relapse suggests device infection and a need to extract the system.
 EPIPHANY	**INPM = DR + GS-BCX + AMT** **PPBC = T4W + AMT** **PNI = SD + AMT**
 DISCUSSION	When to call an Infectious Diseases Consultation: 1) Patients with negative blood cultures and recent prior antibiotics and valve vegetations on TEE should be managed in consultation with an infectious diseases expert. 2) If an infected cardiac device cannot be removed, then long-term suppressive antibiotic therapy should be administered after completing an initial course of treatment and securing a clinical response to therapy. Assess need for reimplantation: reevaluation for continued need of the device should be performed before new device placement. Timing of reimplantation: adequate debridement and control of infection should be achieved at all sites before reimplantation of a new device.
 PEARLS	Skin flora that grows in culture from percutaneous aspirates of fluid or abscess collection should be considered as pathogens. Unlike infective endocarditis, fastidious and uncommon microorganisms that do not grow or stain positive by routinely used laboratory methods have not been identified as pathogens in pacemaker infections. Warning: risk of PE during device extraction from the vegetations.
 REFERENCE	1) Sohail MR, et al. Management and Outcome of Permanent Pacemaker and Implantable Cardioverter-Defibrillator Infections. *J Am Coll Cardiol.* 2007;49;1851–1859. 2) Baddour LM, et al. Nonvalvular Cardiovascular Device–Related Infections. *Circulation.* 2003;108;2015–2031.

CARDIAC DISEASES

Does my patient have amyloid cardiomyopathy?

KEY CONCEPT	The diagnosis of amyloid cardiomyopathy is based on symptomatology, echocardiogram findings, and tissue biopsy.
HISTORY	HPI: Dyspnea, fatigue, syncope. PMH: AL (primary) amyloidosis. FH: Familial amyloidosis.
PHYSICAL EXAM	Peripheral edema, hepatomegaly, hypotension, elevated jugular venous pressure, periorbital purpura.
ELECTRO-CARDIOGRAM	Low voltage, atrial fibrillation.
IMAGING	ECHO: Granular sparkling appearance of myocardium, thickened left ventricle, thickened and dilated right ventricle, mitral and aortic valve leaflet thickening.
SYNTHESIS	**AC** = **A**myloid **C**ardiomyopathy. **SYMP** = **SYMP**toms of dyspnea, fatigue, and/or syncope. **ECHO** = **ECHO**cardiogram findings of granular sparkling myocardium, thickened left and right ventricular, mitral and aortic valve leaflet thickening. **NCARD-BX** = **N**on-**CARD**iac tissue and/or (abdominal fat pad, rectum, or kidney) **B**iopsy positive for amyloid deposits. **IN-NCARD-BX** = **IN**conclusive **N**on-**CARD**iac tissue **B**iopsy. **CARD-BX** = Endomyo**CARD**ial **B**iopsy positive for amyloid deposits.
EPIPHANY	**SYMP + ECHO + NCARD-BX = AC** **SYMP + ECHO + IN-NCARD-BX + CARD-BX = AC**

DISCUSSION	Cardiac amyloidosis should be ruled out in any patient with unexplained heart failure and increased wall thickness on echocardiogram, especially if other clues are present, such as unexplained renal dysfunction or atrial fibrillation.
PEARLS	– Endomyocardial biopsy is virtually 100% sensitive in amyloid cardiomyopathy as amyloid will be deposited all throughout the heart. – In patients with known amyloid deposits in other organs and a history of hypertension, there may be uncertainty as to whether ventricular thickening represents amyloid infiltration or hypertensive heart disease. In such cases, a biopsy may be helpful to determine whether patient has AC.
REFERENCE	1) Falk RH. Diagnosis and Management of the Cardiac Amyloidosis. *Circulation*. 2005;112:2047–2060.

How do I manage my patient with atypical angina (cardiac syndrome X)?

KEY CONCEPT	The management of cardiac syndrome X is based upon pain relief with medication and risk factor reduction.
HISTORY	HPI: Chest pain/discomfort precipitated by exercise or at rest lasting average of 10 minutes. PMH: Hypertension, hyperlipidemia, diabetes. SH: Alcohol, smoking.
ELECTRO-CARDIOGRAM	ECG: Normal findings; ST-segment depression.
IMAGING	Coronary angiogram: Normal. Cardiac MRI: Subendocardial perfusion defects.
SYNTHESIS	**RF-RED** = **R**isk **F**actor **RED**uction: smoking, hypertension, hyperlipidemia, cholesterol, obesity, physical inactivity. **ATEN** = **ATEN**olol 100 mg/day for 4 weeks. **AMLO** = **AMLO**dipine 10 mg/day. **NITR** = isosorbide mono**NITR**ate 10 mg BID. **CSX** = **C**ardiac **S**yndrome **X**.
EPIPHANY	**CSX = RF-RED +/− ATEN/AMLO/NITR**

DISCUSSION	Cardiac syndrome X is believed to be caused by microvascular disease, endothelial dysfunction, and enhanced pain perception. Risk factors are obesity, hypertension, dyslipidemia, glucose intolerance, and proinflammatory states. Syndrome x rarely causes myocardial infarction and it has a good prognosis.
PEARLS	– 10–20% of patients with typical angina chest pain have normal coronary angiograms.
REFERENCE	1) Fraker TD, et al. 2007 Chronic Angina Focused Update of the ACC/AHA 2002 Guidelines for the Management of Patients with Chronic Stable Angina. *J Am Coll Cardiol.* 2007;50:2264. 2) Panting JR, et al. Cardiac Syndrome X. *N Engl J Med.* 2002;346: 1948–1953.

How do I manage acute pericarditis?

KEY CONCEPT	The management of acute pericarditis is based on the resolution of pain, inflammation, and if present effusion.
HISTORY	HPI: Sudden onset of sharp chest pain exacerbated by inspiration and relieved by leaning forward. PMH: Rheumatic heart disease, myocardial infarction, lung cancer, systemic lupus erythematosus. PSH: Coronary artery bypass graft.
PHYSICAL EXAM	Pericardial friction rub, paradoxical pulse (nonpalpable radial or brachial pulse during inspiration), distant heart sounds, elevated JVP.
ELECTRO-CARDIOGRAM	Widespread ST elevation and/or PR depression. Cardiac tamponade (sinus tachycardia, low voltage, or electrical alternans [beat to beat QRS variability]). Figure 37–1
IMAGING	ECHO: Pericardial effusion, cardiac tamponade (diastolic collapse of right atrium and right ventricle, swinging of the heart within pericardial effusion).
SYNTHESIS (cont. on next page)	**APC** = Patient with **A**cute **P**eri**C**arditis. **CTAMP** = Patient with **C**ardiac **TAMP**onade. **CT-AD** = **C**onnective **T**issue or **A**utoimmune **D**isease. **RCT** = Patient with Recurrent Pericarditis unresponsive to medical therapy. **PEF20** = **P**ericardial **EF**fusion > **20** mm present on echocardiogram. **PTN** = Suspected **P**urulent, **T**uberculous, or **N**eoplastic pericarditis. **I-C** = **I**buprofen 300 mg Q6 hours and **C**olchicine 0.5 mg BID. **INEFF I-C** = **INEFF**ective response to **I-C**. **GLC** = **GL**uco**C**orticoids: Prednisone 1 mg/kg/day. Give a short course with a taper as inflammation improves.

SYNTHESIS (cont. from previous page)	**PCDS** = Refer patient for **P**eri**C**ar**D**iocente**S**is. **PCT** = Refer patient for **P**eri**C**ar**D**iec**T**omy.
EPIPHANY	**APC = I-C** **APC + INEFF I-C = GLC** **APC + CT-AD = GLC** **APC + CTAMP = PCDS** **APC + PEF20 = PCDS** **APC + PTN = PCDS** **APC + RCT = PCT**
DISCUSSION	Acute pericarditis is initially managed with NSAIDs and colchicine. Steroids (eg, prednisone) are indicated in patients unresponsive to this first-line treatment and those with connective tissue disease or autoimmune pericarditis etiology. Patients with cardiac tamponade, large effusions (>20 mm), or PTN should be referred for pericardiocentesis. Pericardiectomy is reserved for patients with recurrent episodes of pericarditis poorly controlled by medical therapy.
CONTRA-INDICATIONS	– Aortic dissection is a major contraindication to pericardiocentesis. – Relative contraindications to pericardiocentesis include uncorrected coagulopathy, anticoagulant therapy, thrombocytopenia (<50,000/mm³), small, posterior, and loculated effusions.
PEARLS	– Post-pericardiectomy recurrences of pericarditis may occur due to incomplete resection of the pericardium. – In pericarditis associated with an acute myocardial infarction, aspirin 650 mg Q6 hours is preferred over ibuprofen. – Fever, history of oral anticoagulant therapy, pericarditis associated with trauma, myopericarditis, and a large effusion (>20 mm) are associated with a poor prognosis.
REFERENCE	1) Hoit BD. Management of Effusive and Constrictive Pericardial Heart Disease. *Circulation.* 2002;105;2939–2942. 2) Lange RA. Acute Pericarditis. *N Engl J Med.* 2004;351:2195–2202.

How do I manage cardiac tamponade?

KEY CONCEPT	Relief of increased pericardial pressure is the fundamental aspect of acute management of cardiac tamponade.
HISTORY	HPI: Chest pain; tachypnea, dyspnea. PMH: Malignancy (especially metastatic to thorax), autoimmune disorder, thyroid disorder, uremia, pericarditis, chest trauma, recent thoracotomy, tuberculosis.
PHYSICAL EXAM	Tachycardia, hypotension, jugular venous distension, pulsus paradoxus, kussmaul's sign.
ELECTRO-CARDIOGRAM	Low voltage, sinus tachycardia, electrical alternans (beat to beat QRS variability).
IMAGING	Chest x-ray: Enlarged cardiac silhouette, especially if much larger than prior xrays. Echocardiogram: Best way to rapidly confirm diagnosis as pericardial fluid can be directly visualized and can assess for evidence of tamponade physiology. Also very helpful for treatment planning and during pericardial drainage. CT chest: Pericardial effusions often appear exaggerated on routine non-gated CT scans due to cardiac motion during acquisition.
SYNTHESIS	**CTP** = Patient with diagnosis of **C**ardiac **T**am**P**onade on echocardiogram. **REC** = Patient with **REC**urrent pericardial effusion after being drained before. **PCDS** = Refer patient for **P**eri**C**ar**D**iocente**S**is **PW** = Refer patient for **P**ericardial **W**indow or pericardial stripping. **MED-TX** = Medical management. While waiting for pericardial drainage it is imperative not to diurese the patient, which will drop preload and can precipitate cardiovascular collapse. Start IV fluids and run continuously until pericardial pressure is relieved. When pericardial fluid is obtained send diagnostic studies to identify etiology such as culture, cytology, and adenosine deaminase. If pericardial window or stripping is performed a pericardial biopsy can be obtained. A pericardial drain is usually left in place to drain residual fluid and will need to be removed soon to prevent infectious pericarditis.

E EPIPHANY	**CTP = PCDS + MED-TX** **REC + CTP = PCDS + PW + MED-TX**
DISCUSSION	Pericardiocentesis is best done with imaging to determine which approach (apical or sub-xyphoid) offers the best access to the fluid.
CONTRA- INDICATIONS	Do not diurese patients with cardiac tamponade while they are awaiting drainage!
PEARLS	Echocardiography is the best way to diagnose and plan drainage strategy in cardiac tamponade.
REFERENCE	1) Seferovic MB, et al. Guidelines on the diagnosis and management of pericardial diseases executive summary; The task force on the diagnosis and management of pericardial diseases of the European Society of Cardiology. *Eur Heart J.* 2004;25:387. 2) Spodick DH. Acute Cardiac Tampondae. *N Engl J Med.* 2003;349:684–690.

What should I do if I suspect aortic dissection?

KEY CONCEPT	The initial management of a patient with suspected aortic dissection (AD) is based upon stabilizing the patients BP and heart rate, and selecting the appropriate imaging modality to determine if AD is present.
HISTORY	HPI: Classically sharp, tearing chest pain radiating to the back. Can cause symptoms/signs associated with any of the following due to extension of the dissection: aortic regurgitation, cardiac tamponade, myocardial infarction, stroke, hemorrhagic shock. PMH: peripheral vascular disease, collagen vascular disease, vasculitis, syphilis, bicuspid aortic valve. PSH: Aortic valve replacement. Recent CABG or cardiac catheterization. FH: Marfan's syndrome, Ehlers-Danlos syndrome. SH: Smoking, cocaine.
PHYSICAL EXAM	Diastolic decrescendo murmur, >20 mm Hg variation in systolic BP between both arm, paradoxical pulse (nonpalpable radial or brachial pulse during inspiration).
ELECTRO-CARDIOGRAM	Nonspecific ST and T wave changes. Can be normal or show acute myocardial infarction.
IMAGING	**Transesophageal echocardiogram (TEE):** Can visualize thoracic aorta, aortic root, and aortic valve. Advantage: no radiation and no nephrotoxic contrast required. Can be done at bedside in ICU/CCU if very difficult to transport patient. Disadvantage: cannot visualize abdominal aorta. **CT scan:** Can visualize entire aorta. Advantage: Rapid test, available in most emergency departments. Can see entire dissection and what branches are involved. Disadvantage: Radiation and nephrotoxic contrast used. **MRI:** Similar to CT in capability but more expensive and takes much longer to acquire images.
SYNTHESIS (cont. on next page)	**SAD** = Patient with **S**uspected **A**ortic **D**issection based on clinical presentation. **HU** = **H**emodynamically **U**nstable: hypotension (systolic BP <90 mm Hg) or evidence of shock (mental status changes or decreased urine output). **HS** = **H**emodynamically **S**table: normotensive, normal mentation, no evidence of shock. **STAB** = **STAB**ilize: As quickly as possible, determine if hypotension is due to cardiac tamponade, hemorrhagic shock, or acute myocardial infarction and treat. **IMAGE** = Obtain diagnostic imaging as soon as possible to confirm diagnosis of AD and type. Can use TEE, CT, or MRI depending on institution strengths and availability.

SYNTHESIS (cont. from previous page)	**MED-TX** = Medical management. Goal is to reduced heart rate and blood pressure to reduce shear force that can extend dissection. Admit to intensive care. Pain control with morphine. Keep HR <60 with IV beta blockade (labetalol 20 mg IV q10 min up to 300 mg max), verapamil second line. Keep SBP 100–120 mm Hg (IV betablockade first line, can add nitroprusside 0.5 mcg/kg/min and titrate up to 3 mcg/kg/min). **AD** = **A**ortic **D**issection confirmed by imaging. **CVS** = Consult **C**ardio/**V**ascular **S**urgery. Type-A dissections (involves ascending aorta) are a surgical emergency and CVS should be called emergently. Type-B dissections (does not involve ascending aorta) are usually manage medically but may need operation if there is ongoing hemorrhage. Call CVS emergently if patient unstable.
EPIPHANY	**SAD + HU = STAB + IMAGE** **SAD + HS = IMAGE + MED-TX** **AD + HU = CTS + STAB** **AD + HS = CTS + MED-TX**
DISCUSSION	In patients with suspected AD, blood pressure should be controlled to reduce the shear stress on the aortic wall in order to prevent propagation of a possible dissection and aortic rupture.
CONTRA-INDICATIONS	Do not use medicines that will decrease afterload but not cardiac contractility as this will increase the shear force and can worsen the dissection (ex. hydralazine).
PEARLS	– Stabilize patients first. Then confirm diagnosis with imaging. Medical management can be started in stable patients while awaiting imaging.
REFERENCE	1) Erbel R, et al. Diagnosis and Management of Aortic Dissection: Recommendations of the European Society of Cardiology. *Eur Heart J.* 2001;22:1642–1681. 2) Nienhaber CA, et al. Aortic Dissection: New Frontiers in Diagnosis and Management. *Circulation.* 2003;108:628–635.

How do I manage a patient with aortic dissection?

KEY CONCEPT	The decision to manage a patient with aortic dissection medically or surgically is based on location of dissection and complications.
HISTORY	HPI: Classically sharp, tearing chest pain radiating to the back. Can cause symptoms/signs associated with any of the following due to extension of the dissection: aortic regurgitation, cardiac tamponade, myocardial infarction, stroke, hemorrhagic shock. PMH: peripheral vascular disease, collagen vascular disease, vasculitis, syphilis, bicuspid aortic valve. PSH: Aortic valve replacement. Recent CABG or cardiac catheterization. FH: Marfan's syndrome, Ehlers-Danlos syndrome. SH: Smoking, cocaine.
PHYSICAL EXAM	Diastolic decrescendo murmur, > 20 mm Hg variation in systolic BP between both arm, paradoxical pulse (nonpalpable radial or brachial pulse during inspiration).
ELECTRO-CARDIOGRAM	Nonspecific ST and T wave changes. Can be normal or show acute myocardial infarction.
IMAGING	X-ray: Mediastinal widening, pleural effusion. ECHO: Intimal flap, true and false lumen, thrombosis of false lumen, ascending aortic diameter > 5 cm, aortic regurgitation, pericardial effusion.
SYNTHESIS (cont. on next page)	**SA-AD** = **S**tanford type **A** ascending **A**ortic **D**issection [dissection involving ascending aorta]. This is a surgical emergency and patients are at serious risk as extension of the dissection can compromise the carotid arteries, the coronary arteries, the aortic valve, and the pericardial space. **SB-AD** = **S**tanford type **B A**ortic **D**issection [dissection not involving the descending aorta]. These are usually managed medically unless there is a severe aneurysm with impending rupture or ongoing hemorrhage. **HU** = **H**emodynamically **U**nstable: hypotension (systolic BP < 90 mm Hg) or evidence of shock (mental status changes or decreased urine output). **HS** = **H**emodynamically **S**table: normotensive, normal mentation, no evidence of shock. **STAB** = **STAB**ilize: As quickly as possible, determine if hypotension is due to cardiac tamponade, hemorrhagic shock, or acute myocardial infarction and treat. **MED-TX** = Medical management. Goal is to reduced heart rate and blood pressure to reduce shear force that can extend dissection. Admit to intensive care. Pain control with morphine. Keep HR < 60 with IV beta blockade (labetalol 20 mg IV q10 min up to 300 mg max), verapamil second line. Keep SBP 100–120 mm Hg (IV betablockade first line, can add nitroprusside 0.5 mcg/kg/min and titrate up to 3 mcg/kg/min).

SYNTHESIS (cont. from previous page)	**CVS** = Consult **C**ardio/**V**ascular **S**urgery. Type-A dissections (involves ascending aorta) are a surgical emergency and CVS should be called emergently. Type-B dissections (does not involve ascending aorta) are usually manage medically but may need operation if there is ongoing hemorrhage. Call CVS emergently if patient unstable. If there is a type B dissection and the patient is stable with no evidence of active complication, the patient will still need serial imaging in outpatient follow up to monitor for progression.
E EPIPHANY	**SA-AD + HU = STAB + CVS** **SA-AD + HS = CVS + MED-TX** **SB-AD + HU = STAB + CVS** **SB-AD + HS = MED-TX + CVS**
DISCUSSION	In patients with aortic dissection, blood pressure should be controlled to reduce the shear stress on the aortic wall in order to prevent propagation of a possible dissection and aortic rupture.
CONTRA-INDICATIONS	– Do not use medicines that will decrease afterload but not cardiac contractility as this will increase the shear force and can worsen the dissection (ex. hydralazine).
PEARLS	– Type-A dissections (involves ascending aorta) are a surgical emergency and CVS should be called emergently.
REFERENCE	1) Erbel R, et al. Diagnosis and Management of Aortic Dissection. *Eur Heart J.* 2001;22:1642–1648.

How do I manage my patient with a left ventricular thrombus?

KEY CONCEPT	The management of a left ventricular thrombus (LVT) is focused at preventing thromboembolism such as stroke.
HISTORY	HPI: LVT detected on echocardiogram. PMH: Myocardial infarction, coronary artery disease, AFIB, dilated cardiomyopathy, ischemic stroke. PSH: Alcohol, smoking.
ELECTRO-CARDIOGRAM	ST elevation especially in V4-V5 (anterior leads) indicating old ventricular aneurysm.
IMAGING	**ECHO:** Direct visualization of intracardiac thrombus (sensitivity improved with echocontrast), regional or global wall motion abnormalities, left ventricular aneurysm. **Cardiac MRI:** Very sensitive and specific for chronic LV thrombus.
SYNTHESIS	**LVT = L**eft **V**entricular **T**hrombus detected (ex. on echocardiogram.) **LV-SC = L**eft **V**entricular **S**tructural **C**hange: severe hypokinesis/akinesis/dyskinesis of the left ventricle (especially near apex). Left ventricular aneurysm formation. **AC = A**nti**C**oagulation: Must ensure there is no significant contraindication to anticoagulation before initiating. Can use warfarin initiated at 5 mg/day and titrated to target INR of 2.0–3.0. Anticoagulate patients for a minimum of 3 months. If there is no increased risk of bleeding, continue anticoagulation for life. **FOLLOW =** Follow up: obtain a repeat echocardiogram in 3–6 months to assess for resolution or evolution of the thrombus.
EPIPHANY	**LVT = AC + FOLLOW** **LVT + LV-SC = AC + FOLLOW**

DISCUSSION	Development of a left ventricular thrombus is a common complication of a myocardial infarction and can lead to an embolic stroke if not treated correctly. Anticoagulation appears to reduce the incidence of embolization even if thrombus remains on repeat echocardiogram. High risk features for embolization are very mobile thrombi and long thrombi that protrude into the LV cavity. There are no hard and fast guidelines on how to manage these patients. Risk versus benefit must be weighed individually for patients. Patients with permanent wall motion abnormality (particularly at the apex) or aneurysm in the setting of severely depressed LV function will probably remain at increased risk for LVT for life. It is reasonable to anticoagulate these patients even before a diagnosis of LVT is made.
PEARLS	– Anticoagulation appears to reduce the incidence of embolization even if thrombus remains on repeat echocardiogram.
REFERENCE	1) Antman EM, et al. 2007 Focused Update of the ACC/AHA 2004 Guidelines for the Management of Patients with ST-Elevation Myocardial Infarction. *J Am Coll Cardiol*. 2008;51;210–247.

Does my pregnant patient have peripartum cardiomyopathy?

KEY CONCEPT	The diagnosis of peripartum cardiomyopathy (PPCM) is based upon clinical findings and imaging.
HISTORY	HPI: Dyspnea, cough, fatigue, chest discomfort, orthopnea, hemoptysis, abdominal pain, arrhythmias, thromboembolism, asymptomatic LV dysfunction. FH: PPCM.
PHYSICAL EXAM	ECHO: Left ventricular ejection fraction (LVEF) <45%, left ventricular enlargement.
SYNTHESIS	**PPCM** = **P**eri**P**artum **C**ardio**M**yopathy. **CF** = Development of **C**ardiac **F**ailure in the last month of pregnancy or within 5 months of delivery. **ABS-IC** = **ABS**ence of an **I**dentifiable **C**ause for the cardiac failure, and high suspicion of nonischemic cardiomyopathy. **ABS-RHD** = **ABS**ence of **R**ecognizable **H**eart **D**isease prior to the last month of pregnancy. **LVSD** = **L**eft **V**entricular **S**ystolic **D**ysfunction (LVEF <45%).
EPIPHANY	**CF + ABS-IC + ABS-RHD + LVSD = PPCM**
DISCUSSION	Once a patient is diagnosed with PPCM, treatment should be begun to alleviate symptoms of heart failure. Treatment: Safe drugs = Digoxin, nitrates, hydralazine, heparin, diuretics, beta-blockers. Taken till LV EF normalizes. Unsafe drugs = ACEI, nitroprusside, coumadin, amiodarone.

PEARLS	– Risk factors for PPCM are multiparity, advanced maternal age, multifetal pregnancy, preeclampsia, and gestational hypertension. – Subsequent pregnancy can lead to persistent depression of LVEF, CHF, and even death.
REFERENCE	1) Pearson GD, et al. Peripartum Cardiomyopathy. *JAMA*. 2000;283(9): 1183–1188.

How do I diagnose a patient with deep venous thrombosis?

KEY CONCEPT	In patients with deep venous thrombosis (DVT), the diagnosis is based upon clinical suspicion and imaging findings.
HISTORY	HPI: Discomfort and pain in calf, recent immobilization for prolonged period of time. PMH: Obesity, antithrombin deficiency, protein C or S deficiency, Factor V Leiden mutation. PSH: Recent hospitalization for surgery.
PHYSICAL EXAM	Palpable cord; ipsilateral edema, warmth, and/or superficial venous dilation; Homan's sign (dorsiflexion of the foot elicits pain in the posterior calf), Pratt's sign (squeezing of posterior calf elicits pain).
IMAGING	Compression ultrasonography: Abnormal compressibility of vein, abnormal Doppler color flow, presence of echogenic band.
SYNTHESIS	**DVT** = **D**eep **V**ein **T**hrombosis. **NO-DVT** = **NO D**eep **V**ein **T**hrombosis. **CLIN** = **CLIN**ical findings: patient complaining of discomfort and pain in calf, or physical exam findings of pain, tenderness, and swelling in leg. **COMP-US** = **COMP**ression **U**ltra**S**onography with findings of: abnormal compressibility of vein; abnormal Doppler color flow; presence of echogenic band. **INCON** = **INCON**clusive. **VENO-POS** = **VENO**graphy **POS**itive for DVT. **VENO-NEG** = **VENO**graphy **NEG**ative for DVT.
EPIPHANY	**CLIN + COMP-US = DVT** **CLIN + INCON[COMP-US] + VENO-POS = DVT** **CLIN + INCON[COMP-US] + VENO-NEG = NO-DVT**
DISCUSSION	In patients with DVT, prompt diagnosis and treatment are essential to prevent the occurrence of a pulmonary embolism. The low incidence of factor V Leiden and prothrombin G20210A may not warrant aggressive prophylaxis or genetic testing until a second event occurs.

PEARLS	For isolated deep-vein thrombosis in the calf, the sensitivity of ultrasonography is lower, and thus contrast venography is preferred if clinical suspicion is high.
REFERENCE	1) Jaff MR, et al. Management of Massive and Submassive Pulmonary Embolism, Iliofemoral Deep Venous Thrombosis, and Chronic Thromboembolic Pulmonary Hypertension. *Circulation*. 2011;123:1788–1830. 2) Hirsch J, et al. Management of Deep Vein Thrombosis and Pulmonary Embolism. *Circulation*. 1996;93:2212–2245. 3) Bates SM, et al. Treatment of Deep-Vein Thrombosis. *N Engl J Med*. 2004;351:268–277.

How do I manage a patient with deep venous thrombosis?

KEY CONCEPT	In patients with deep venous thrombosis (DVT), the management is based upon relief of symptoms, prevention of embolization, and recurrence with anticoagulation.
HISTORY	HPI: Discomfort and pain in calf. PMH: Obesity, antithrombin deficiency, protein C or S deficiency, Factor V Leiden mutation. PSH: Recent hospitalization for surgery.
PHYSICAL EXAM	Homan's sign (dorsiflexion of the foot elicits pain in the posterior calf), Pratt's sign (squeezing of posterior calf elicits pain).
IMAGING	Compression ultrasonography: Abnormal compressibility of vein, abnormal Doppler color flow, presence of echogenic band.
SYNTHESIS	**DVT** = **D**eep **V**enous **T**hrombosis. **APDVT/APE** = **A**cute **P**roximal **DVT** or **A**cute **P**ulmonary **E**mbolism. **HIT** = **H**eparin **I**nduced **T**hrombocytopenia (suspected or proven). **ENOX** = **ENOX**aparin 1 mg/kg every 12 hours subcutaneously, maximum of 180 mg/day. APTT goal of 1.5 times upper limit of normal (45 seconds). Continue for minimum of 5 days, and/or discontinue when INR is >=2.0 for at least 24 hours (target INR is 2.0–3.0). **UNFH** = **UNF**ractionated **H**eparin 80 U/kg bolus followed by a continuous infusion, initially at 18 U/kg/hr (dose adjust to goal APTT 1.5–2.3 times control (46–70 seconds). Continue for minimum of 5 days, and/or discontinue when INR is >=2.0 for at least 24 hours (target INR is 2.0–3.0). **FOND** = **FOND**aparinux subcutaneous injection once daily: 5 mg for patients 50 kg weight, 7.5 mg for 50–100, and 10 mg for >100 kg. Discontinue when INR is within therapeutic range of 2–3. **COUM** = **COUM**adin initiated at 5 mg/day, and titrated for target INR of 2.0–3.0. Continue for 3 months (in patients with first-episode of DVT related to a major reversible risk factor), 6 months (patients with recurrent or unprovoked DVT). **DTI** = **D**irect **T**hrombin **I**nhibitor (see chapter on DTI). **CI-AC** = **C**ontra**I**ndication to **A**nti**C**oagulation (active bleeding; platelet count <20000/mm³; neurosurgery, ocular surgery or intracranial bleeding within past 10 days). **INEFF-AC** = If **A**nti**C**oagulation with ENOX,UNFH or FOND and COUM is **INEFF**ective. **IVCF** = Refer patient for **I**nferior **V**ena **C**ava **F**ilter placement.

 EPIPHANY	**DVT = ENOX + COUM** or 　　　**UNFH + COUM** or 　　　**FOND + COUM** **DVT + HIT = DTI + COUM** **APDVT/APE + CI-AC = IVCF** **APDVT/APE + INEFF-AC = IVCF**
 DISCUSSION	In patients with DVT, prompt diagnosis and treatment are essential to prevent the formation of a pulmonary embolism. To reduce hospital length of stay, begin enoxaparin and coumadin at the same time.
 PEARLS	Low-molecular-weight heparin (enoxaparin) has a lower risk of heparin-induced thrombocytopenia than unfractionated heparin as well as a greater bioavailability when given by subcutaneous injection. In cancer patients with DVT, treat with ENOX monotherapy for 3–6 months, or as long as cancer or treatment is ongoing.
 REFERENCE	1) Jaff MR, et al. Management of Massive and Submassive Pulmonary Embolism, Iliofemoral Deep Venous Thrombosis, and Chronic Thromboembolic Pulmonary Hypertension. *Circulation*. 2011;123:1788–1830. 2) Bates SM, et al. Treatment of Deep-Vein Thrombosis. *N Engl J Med*. 2004;351:268–277. 3) Kahn SR, et al. Therapy for Venous Thromboembolic Disease. *Chest*. 2008;133:454S–545S.

How do I diagnose pulmonary embolism in my patient?

KEY CONCEPT	The diagnosis of pulmonary embolism (PE) can sometimes be difficult and is based up on clinical suspicion and diagnostic testing.
HISTORY	HPI: Dyspnea, chest pain, cough, hemoptysis, recent trauma/surgery, smoking, pregnancy, hormone contraceptive/therapy Labs: PT/PTT, Troponin, BNP, creatinine, d-dimer PMH: Obesity, hypercoaguable state, history of DVT or PE, malignancy
PHYSICAL EXAM	Resp: Hypoxia, tachypnea, hemoptysis. CV: Tachycardia, hypotension. Ext: Leg swelling.
IMAGING	ECG: RV strain, S1T3Q3, sinus tachycardia, Q in III, aVF, right axis deviation, RBBB. Echocardiogram: Right ventricular dysfunction and akinesia. V/Q scan: Perfusion defect. CT angiogram: Filling defect, RV dilation.
SYNTHESIS	**PE** = **P**ulmonary **E**mbolism **NO-PE** = Insufficient evidence to make the diagnosis of PE. Modified Wells Criteria: Clinical symptoms of DVT (3 points), Other diagnoses less likely than PE (3 points), Heart rate >100 (1.5 points), Immobilization ≥3 days or surgery in previous four weeks (1.5 points), Previous DVT/PE (1.5 points), Hemoptysis (1 point), Malignancy (1 point) **W-UNLIKELY** = Wells Score =< 4 **W-LIKELY** = Wells Score > 4. Must obtain further testing such as CT Angiogram to affirm or exclude PE. **DD-NEG** = D-Dimer level < 500 ng/mL **DD-POS** = D-Dimer level > 500 ng/mL **CTA-NEG** = **CT A**ngio **NEG**ative for PE. Like any test, a CT angiogram is not 100% sensitive and specific. Rarely the test is non-diagnostic or the clinical suspicion is still too high to exclude PE, and a pulmonary angiogram can be done. **CTA-POS** = **CT A**ngiogram **POS**itive for PE.
EPIPHANY	**W-UNLIKELY + DD-NEG = NO-PE (no further testing)** **W-LIKELY + DD-NEG/POS + CTA-POS = PE** **W-LIKELY + DD-NEG/POS + CTA-NEG = NO-PE**

 DISCUSSION	Pulmonary embolism can be an elusive diagnosis that results in considerable morbidity and mortality. Patients present in a variety of ways many of the signs and symptoms are nonspecific. Think about pulmonary embolism in your patients, especially when something "doesn't fit" the clinical picture such as unexplained tachycardia or fever.
 PEARLS	A very low D-dimer level has a high negative predictive value and can safely exclude the presence of pulmonary embolism without further testing when the pre-test probability is low.
 REFERENCE	1) Torbicki A, et al. Guidelines on the Diagnosis and Management of Acute Pulmonary Embolism: The Task Force for the Diagnosis and Management of Acute Pulmonary Embolism of the European Society of Cardiology (ESC). *Eur Heart J.* 2008;29:2276–2315. 2) Goldhaber SZ, Visani L, De Rosa M. Acute Pulmonary Embolism: Clinical Outcomes in the International Cooperative Pulmonary Embolism Registry (ICOPER). *Lancet.* 1999;353:1386–1389.

How do I treat my patient with acute pulmonary embolism?

 KEY CONCEPT	In patients with pulmonary embolism (PE) the management is based upon relief of symptoms prevention of recurrence of disease with anticoagulation and in severe cases removal of the clot.
 HISTORY	HPI: SOB, chest pain, cough, hemoptysis, age >50, recent trauma/surgery, smoking, pregnancy. Labs: PT/PTT, troponin, BNP, creatinine, D-dimer. PMH: Obesity, antithrombin deficiency, protein C/S deficiency, Factor V Leiden mutation, presence or history of DVT, malignancy, hormone contraceptive/therapy. PSH: Recent hospitalization for surgery, prolonged immobilization.
 PHYSICAL EXAM	Resp: Hypoxia, tachypnea, hemoptysis. CV: Tachycardia, hypotension. Ext: Leg swelling.
 IMAGING	ECG: RV strain, S1T3Q3, sinus tachycardia, Q in III, aVF, right axis deviation, RBBB. Echocardiogram: Right ventricular dysfunction, akinesia, RVSP >40 mm Hg. V/Q scan: Perfusion defect. CT angiogram: Filling defect, RV dilation.
SYNTHESIS (cont. on next page)	**PE** = Patient diagnosed with acute **P**ulmonary **E**mbolism. **HEP** = Unfractionated IV **HEP**arin (bolus of 80 U/kg followed by continuous infusion dosed at 18 U/kg/hr with dose adjustment). **ENOX** = **ENOX**aparin 1 mg/kg every 12 hours subcutaneously, maximum of 180 mg/day. APTT goal of 1.5 times upper limit of normal (45 seconds). Discontinue when INR is therapeutic range of 2–3 if bridging with Coumadin. **COUM** = **COUM**adin 5 mg/day with target INR of 2–3. Continue for 3–6 months for first PE, lifetime for second PE with INR 2.5–3.5. **THROM** = **THROM**bolysis for massive PE with hemodynamic compromise or RV dysfunction (streptokinase 250,000-IU IV bolus followed by100,000-IU/hr infusion for 12–24 hours or alteplase 100 mg IV infusion over 2 hours). **UNSTABLE** = Hypotension, shock, SBP <90 mm Hg, drop of 40 mm Hg, respiratory distress. **CI-THROM** = **C**ontra**I**ndication to **THROM**bolysis. **INEFF-THROM** = **INEFF**ective **THROM**bolysis. **CI-AC** = **C**ontra**I**ndication to **A**nti**C**oagulation (active bleeding; platelet count <20,000/mm³; neurosurgery, ocular surgery, or intracranial bleeding within past 10 days).

SYNTHESIS (cont. from previous page)	**INEFF-AC** = If **A**nti**C**oagulation with ENOX and COUM is **INEFF**ective or recurrent PE. **IVCF** = Refer patient for **I**nferior **V**ena **C**ava **F**ilter placement. **SURG** = Refer patient for **SURG**ical embolectomy/endarterectomy.
EPIPHANY	**PE = ENOX/HEP + COUM** **PE + CI-AC = IVCF** **PE + INEFF-AC = IVCF** **PE + UNSTABLE = THROM** **PE + UNSTABLE + CI-THROM = SURG**
DISCUSSION	In patients with PE, prompt diagnosis and treatment are essential to prevent cardiorespiratory failure and sudden cardiac death. An abnormal D-dimer level at the end of therapy may signal the need of continue treatment in patients with first PE. If untreated, mortality is as high as 26%. If the patient has contraindication to LMWH (kidney failure) then admission to hospital is needed for bridging with IV unfractionated heparin.
PEARLS	– Low-molecular-weight heparin may reduce bleeding compared to unfractionated heparin in patients with PE. It also has a lower risk of heparin-induced thrombocytopenia as well as a greater bioavailability when given by subcutaneous injection. – Avoid Coumadin in pregnant patients.
REFERENCE	1) Bates SM, et al. Treatment of Deep-Vein Thrombosis. *N Engl J Med* 2004;351:268–277. 2) Kahn SR, et al. Therapy for Venous Thromboembolic Disease. *Chest.* 2008;133:454S–545S. Goldhaber SZ. Pulmonary embolism. *Lancet.* 2004;363(9417):1295. 3) Barritt DW, Jordan SC. Anticoagulant Drugs in the Treatment of Pulmonary Embolism: A Controlled Trial. *Lancet.* 1960;1(7138):1309–1312. 4) Torbicki A, et al. Guidelines on the Diagnosis and Management of Acute Pulmonary Embolism: The Task Force for the Diagnosis and Management of Acute Pulmonary Embolism of the European Society of Cardiology (ESC). *Eur Heart J.* 2008;29:2276–2315.

Does my patient have pheochromocytoma?

KEY CONCEPT	The diagnosis of pheochromocytoma is based upon presence of symptoms and presence of urinary catecholamines and metanephrines.
HISTORY	HPI: Palpitations, headache, sweating, generalized weakness. PMH: Von Hippel–Lindau syndrome (hemangioblastoma of brain and spine, retinal angioma, tumors of the middle ear), neurofibromatosis type 1 (café au lait spots, axillary and inguinal freckling, and iris hamartomas), hyperparathyroidism, medullary thyroid cancer. FH: Multiple endocrine neoplasia type 2A (medullary thyroid cancer, pheochromocytoma, parathyroid hyperplasia).
ELECTRO-CARDIOGRAM	Tachycardia.
SYNTHESIS	**PHEO** = Patient has **PHEO**chromocytoma. **PHEO-SYMP** = Triad of SYMPtoms of palpitations, headache, and sweating. **URIN-POS** = 24-hour **URIN**ary catecholamine and metanephrine test is **POS**itive (norepinephrine > 170 mcg/24 hr, epinephrine > 5 mcg/24 hr, dopamine > 700 mcg/24 hr, or metanephrine > 400 mcg/24 hr).
E EPIPHANY	**PHEO-SYMP + URIN-POS = PHEO**
DISCUSSION	Pheochromocytoma is rare but important diagnosis to be considered in the evaluation of patients with hypertension, arrhythmias, and panic disorder and in the follow-up of particular genetic disease.

 PEARLS	– Tricyclic antidepressants most commonly interfere with interpretation of 24-hour urinary catecholamine and metanephrine testing and should be tapered and discontinued for at least 2 weeks prior to diagnostic testing.
 REFERENCE	1) Young WF Jr. Pheochromocytoma: 1926–1993. In *Trends in Endocrinology and Metabolism*, Vol. 4, p. 122. Elsevier Science, Inc.; 1993. 2) Pacak K, et al. Recent Advances in Genetics, Diagnosis, Localization, and Treatment of Pheochromocytoma. *Ann Intern Med.* 2001;134(4): 315–329.

How do I manage a patient with pheochromcytoma?

KEY CONCEPT	Pheochromocytoma is a condition where the adrenal gland secrets excess catecholamines, causing elevated blood pressures and heart rates as well as sympathetic overactivity.
HISTORY	Patients will present with skin sensation (flushing, diaphoresis, sweating), tachycardia, paroxysmal hypertension, anxiety, headaches.
PHYSICAL EXAM	Paroxysmal hypertension, tachycardia, arrhythmias, orthostatic hypotension, papilledema, polyuria, hyperglycemia, leukocytosis.
ELECTRO-CARDIOGRAM	T wave inversions, sinus tachycardia, LVH.
IMAGING	ECHO: LVH, tachycardia-induced cardiomyopathy, wall motion abnormalities, dilated cardiomyopathy. CT scan with contrast. T2-weighted MRI. MIBG scintigraphy. PET scan.
SYNTHESIS	**U-HTN** = **U**ncontrolled **H**yper**T**ensio**N**. **I-HTN** = **I**nadequately controlled BP despite labetolol or contraindication to labetolol. **PT** = **P**oor **T**olerance to standard medications. **S** = **S**urgery (definitive treatment of choice). **METS** = Metastatic lesions, surgery not an option. **A-HTN** = **A**cute **H**yper**T**ensive crisis. **LAB** = **LAB**etalol 40–80 mg IV q10 minutes. **NIC** = Nicardipie 5 mg/hr and titrate 2.5 mg/hr q5–15 min prn. **MET** = Metyrosine 250 mg QID PO. **PRES** = Preoperative preparation via blood **PRES**sure control (phenoxybenzamine 10 mg x 1 week) and salt load (5000 mg daily) to prevent post-surgical hypotension. **ALPHA** = **ALPHA** blockers—prazosin 1 mg TID max 15 mg. **IV-MEDS** = Sodium nitroprusside 0.25 mcg/kg/min and titrate, nicardipine, phentolamine bolus (1–5 mg).

E EPIPHANY	**U-HTN = LAB** **I-HTN = NIC** **I-HTN + PT = MET** **S = PRES** **METS = ALPHA** **A-HTN = IV-MEDS**
DISCUSSION	– Suspect pheochromocytoma if hypertension is resistant to traditional medications. – The classic triad is headache, sweating, tachycardia.
PEARLS	Avoid beta blockers (may worsen blood pressure). Caution salt load in patients with CHF/renal failure.
REFERENCE	1) Gifford RW Jr. Management of Hypertensive Crises. *JAMA*. 1991; 266–829. 2) Kassin TA, Clarke DD, Mi VQ, et al. Catecholamine-Induced Cardiomyopathy. *Endocr Pract*. 2008;14:1137.

How do you manage a patient with myocarditis?

KEY CONCEPT	Myocarditis is a condition where the heart muscle is inflamed and damaged without coronary artery blockage, resulting in a decrease in cardiac function.
HISTORY	Patient with recent infection presents with fever, viral prodromes, chest pain, joint pain, myalgias, fatigue, dyspnea palpitations, or heart failure. Establish characteristics of chest pain, presence of sick contacts, cardiac toxic medications/drugs, cardiac history, family history of cardiac disease.
PHYSICAL EXAM	Fever, signs of diminished cardiac output, tachycardia, weak pulses, cool extremities, muffled heart sounds, presence of S3, JVD, and edema. Ongoing myocardial inflammation may result in dilated cardiomyopathy, restrictive CMP, or acute LV failure without LV dilatation.
ELECTRO- CARDIOGRAM	Diffuse T wave inversions and ST segment elevations. Severe changes could have bundle branch, high-degree AV blocks, and Q waves.
IMAGING	CXR: Cardiomegaly, pulmonary effusion. Echocardiogram evaluates LVEF, chamber size (presence of left ventricular dilation), wall motion abnormalities, increased LV EDV, presence of effusions. Cardiac MRI reveals inflammation, delayed contrast enhancement, following gadolinium infusion and increased T2 signals.
SYNTHESIS	**MYO-U** = Uncomplicated Myocarditis. **MYO-C** = Myocarditis with cardiac dysfunction. **MYO-S** = Myocarditis with severe dysfunction and morbidity. **ST** = **S**upportive **T**herapy (for uncomplicated conditions: symptomatic therapy, best rest, pain control, NSAIDs). **MT** = **M**edical **T**herapy (if cardiac dysfunction is present, use ACEI, inotropes (milrinone), digoxin, diuretics, IVIG, steroids, carvedilol). **UNRES-MT** = Patient **UNRES**ponsive to **M**edical **T**herapy. **EMBX** = **E**ndo**M**yocardial **B**iopsy. **AVT** = **A**nti**V**iral **T**herapy (antiviral therapy with ribavirin/interferon alpha immunosuppressive therapy with corticosteroids, cyclosporine, azathioprine). **UNRES-AVT** = Patient **UNRES**ponsive to **A**nti**V**iral **T**herapy.
EPIPHANY	**MYO-U = ST** **MYO-C = MT** **MOC-C + UNRES-MT = EMBX** **MYO-S = AVT** **MYO-S + UNRES-AVT = EMBX**

 DISCUSSION	– Myocarditis can cause mild disease with self-resolution, chest pain, heart failure, arrhythmias, and sudden cardiac death. – Common causes are virus (coxsackie, parvoirus, EBV, CMV, adenovirus), bacteria (*Borrelia, Brucella, Rickettsia, Haemophilus*), protozoa (trypanosome), fungal (*Aspergillus*) hypersensitivity to drugs, autoimmune reactions, and toxins. – Routine use of immunosuppressive therapy is not recommended in myocarditis. – Endomyocardial biopsy is recommended in patients with acute deterioration of cardiac function of unknown etiology who are unresponsive to medical therapy. Transcriptomic biomarkers from a single endomyocardial biopsy can improve the clinical detection of patients with inflammatory diseases of the heart. This approach advances the clinical management and treatment of cardiac disorders with highly variable outcome.
 PEARLS	– 20% of sudden cardiac deaths are from myocarditis. – Complete recovery of ventricular function is seen is as much as 50% of patients. – Most causes/etiologies are not found; definite diagnosis requires heart muscle biopsy. – Place patient on telemetry/electrocardiographic monitoring. Check CBC, blood cultures, cardiac enzymes (CKMB, troponin I), LDH, serial ECG, Echo, ESR/CRP, IgM serology of viruses and cultures, LFTs, anti-alpha myosin autoantibodies, anti-cardiac IgG.
 REFERENCE	1) Mahrholdt H, et al. Presentation, Patterns of Myocardial Damage, and Clinical Course of Viral Myocarditis. *Circulation*. 2006;114:1581. 2) Gerzen P, et al. Acute Myocarditis. A Follow-up Study. *Br Heart J*. 1972;34:575. 3) Heidecker B, et al. Transcriptomic Biomarkers for the Accurate Diagnosis of Myocarditis. *Circulation*. 2011;123:1174–1184.

EXAMINATION

What are the abnormal pulses in my patient and what cardiac conditions are they associated with?

 KEY CONCEPT	Important information about the patient cardiac status is obtained by physical examination of arterial pulses. A differential diagnosis can be made by inspecting the arterial blood pressure and central/peripheral pulses.
 HISTORY	Patient being evaluated presents with abnormal pulses on physical exam.
 PHYSICAL EXAM	Listen for murmurs, rubs, gallops, location of cardiac impulse, parasternal lifts.
SYNTHESIS	**SWP** = **S**mall **W**eak **P**ulse. **HKP** = **H**ypo**K**inetic **P**ulse. **DP** = **D**elayed **P**ulse. **LBP** = **L**arge **B**ounding **P**ulse. **DPP** = **D**ouble **P**eak **P**ulse **PWSD** = **P**alpable **W**aves: 1 in **S**ystole, 1 in **D**iastole. **AAP** = **A**lteration of **A**mplitude **P**ulse. **DPDI** = **D**ecreased **P**ulse or absent **D**uring **I**nspiration. **SULE** = **S**lower **U**pstroke of **L**ower **E**xtremity pulse compared to upper extremity/disparity in amplitude. **PP** = **P**ulsus **P**arvus (dimished left ventricular stroke volume, narrow pulse pressure, increased peripheral vascular resistance) **HV** = **H**yop**V**olemia **LVF** = **L**eft **V**entricular **F**ailure **RC** = **R**estrictive **C**ardiomyopathy **MS** = **M**itral **S**tenosis **PT** = **P**ulses **T**ardus: aortic stenosis with delayed systolic peak, left ventricular obstruction. **KERKP** = **H**yp**ERK**inetic **P**ulse-increased LV stroke volume, wide pulse pressure, decreased peripheral vascular resistance: AV fi stulas, mitral regurgitation, ventricular septal defect. **BWC** = **B**isferiens/**W**ater hammer/**C**orrigan: aortic regurgitation, hypertrophic cardiomyopathy. **DICR** = **DICR**rotic: low stroke volumes, dilated cardiomyopathy. **PALT** = **P**ulsus **ALT**ernans: severe impairment of LV function. **PPAR** = **P**ulsus paradoxus: tamponade, airway obstruction, superior vena cava obstruction. **RFD** = **R**adio**F**emoral **D**elay: coarcation of aorta.

 EPIPHANY	**SWP = PP** **HKP = HV or LVF or RC or MS** **DP = PT** **LBP = HERKP** **DPP = BWC** **PWSD = DICR** **AAP = PALT** **DPDI = PPAR** **SULE = RFD**
 DISCUSSION	The arterial pulse begins when the aortic valve opens and left ventricle contracts. There is a rapid rise called the anacrotic notch; then during isovolumic relaxation, there is a reversal of flow prior to aortic valve closure which is called the incisura.
 PEARLS	Palpate all pulses and note for any differences between them, as well as do simultaneous palpation of pulses on each side of the body. Palpation of pulses can also give information about heart blocks and irregular rhythms: regular irregular pulses are seen in PAC/PVC, irregular irregular pulses seen in atrial fibrillation.
 REFERENCE	1) Chizner M, ed. *Classic Teachings in Clinical Cardiology: A Tribute to W. Proctor Harvey.* Cedar Grove, NY: Laennec; 1996. 2) Fauci AS, Braunwald E, Isselbacher KJ, et al., eds. *Harrisons Principles of Internal Medicine.* 15th ed. New York, NY: McGraw-Hill; 2007.

What is the likely heart murmur I hear?

KEY CONCEPT	Auscultation of murmurs is reliable and cost effective to make diagnosis of various heart conditions.
HISTORY	Asymptomatic/symptomatic patient with murmur presenting with or without respiratory distress, pallor, cyanosis, clubbing, diaphoresis, chest pain.
PHYSICAL EXAM	Note intensity 1–6 (1 being barely audible, 6 being heard without stethoscope without contact to chest). Note the configuration (crescendo, decrescendo, diamond shaped, plateau), onset and cessation, location, radiation, time during cardiac cycle, and response to maneuvering.
IMAGING	Two-dimensional Echo and color Doppler flow.
SYNTHESIS (cont. on next page)	**Systolic Murmurs:** **MR** = **M**itral **R**egurgitation. **TR** = **T**ricuspid **R**egurgitation. **VSD** = **V**entricular **S**eptal **D**efect. **IM** = **I**nnocent **M**urmur. **AS** = **A**ortic **S**tenosis. **PS** = **P**ulmonic **S**tenosis. **HOCM** = **H**yertrophic **O**bstructive **C**ardio**M**yopathy. **MVP** = **M**itral **V**alve **P**rolapse. **ASD** = **A**trial **S**eptal **D**efect. **CAV** = **C**alcific **A**ortic **V**alve. **HS** = **H**olosystolic. **MDE** = **M**idsystolic **E**jection. **MSM** = **M**id**S**ystolic **M**urmur. **MSC** = **M**id**S**ystolic **C**lick and murmur. **IA** = **I**naudible **A**2. **Diastolic Murmurs:** **AR** = **A**ortic **R**egurgitation. **PR** = **P**ulmonic **R**egurgitation. **MS** = **M**itral **S**tenosis. **TS** = **T**ricuspid **S**tenosis. **ED** = **E**arly **D**iastolic. **MRD** = **M**id-**R**umbling **D**iastolic.

 SYNTHESIS (cont. from previous page)	**Continuous Murmurs:** **PDA** = **P**atent **D**uctus **A**rteriosus. **CONT** = **CONT**inuous venous hum.
 EPIPHANY	MR/TR/VSD = HS IM = MDE AS/PS/HOCM/ASD = MSM MVP = MSC CAV = IA AR/PR = ED MS/TS = MRD PDA = CONT
 DISCUSSION	The presence of murmurs should be taken into the context of the patient with importance of noting presence of known cardiac and symptoms. The approach to the patient should first determine if murmur is systolic or diastolic. Diastolic and continuous murmurs should be evaluated by echocardiogram and cardiac catheterization if appropriate. Systolic murmurs grade 1–2 without symptoms, or other findings do not require further workup. Systolic murmurs 1–2 with symptoms or cardiac findings or grade 3 or higher holosystolic or late should be evaluated with echocardiography.
 PEARLS	All diastolic/holosystolic/late systolic murmurs are pathologic. Early and midsystolic murmurs may be functional. Accentuation during inspiration implies origination on the right side and during expiration implies origination on the left side. Valsalva reduces intensity of most by reducing ventricular filling except MVP and HOCM (which are louder upon standing). Most murmurs are louder following PVC (except regurgitant murmurs).
 REFERENCE	1) Fustr V, O'rourke RA, Walsh RA, et al., eds. *Hurst's The Heart*. 12th ed. New York, NY: McGraw-Hill; 2008. 2) Fauci AS, Braundwald E, Isselbacher KJ, et al., eds. *Harrison's Principles of Internal Medicine*. 15th ed. New York, NY: McGraw-Hill; 2007.

Does my patient need preoperative cardiac testing for noncardiac surgery?

KEY CONCEPT	The decision to perform preoperative cardiac testing for noncardiac surgery is best on underlying cardiac conditions, risk factors, type or procedure, and the patient's functional capacity.
HISTORY	HPI: Patient with underlying cardiac condition undergoing noncardiac surgery. PMH: Coronary artery disease, congestive heart failure, aortic dissection, peripheral artery disease, stroke, diabetes. SH: Smoking, alcohol.
ELECTRO-CARDIOGRAM	ECG: ST-segment elevation, ST-segment depression, deep Q waves (>1 mm), PR interval irregularly variable, narrow QRS complex.
IMAGING	X-ray: Cardiomegaly, cephalization of pulmonary vessels (increased distribution of flow to apices), pleural effusion. ECHO: Left ventricular ejection fraction <40%, left atrial and left ventricular enlargement; mitral valve annular calcification, thickened/calcific aortic valve, bicuspid aortic valve.
SYNTHESIS	**PREOP-PT = PREOP**erative **Pa**Tient, ie, going for surgery. **ACC = A**ctive **C**ardiac **C**ondition: valvular disease; arrhythmia (2nd degree type atrioventricular (AV) block, 3rd degree AV block, ventricular tachycardia, supraventricular tachycardia); decompensated heart failure; recent myocardial infarction (within 30 days); extensive angina (marked limitation of physical activities, angina present at rest, inability to perform activity without discomfort). **E-T = E**valuate condition and **T**reat condition prior to surgery. **HRP = H**igh-**R**isk **P**rocedure: aortic or major vascular surgery; peripheral arterial surgery; cardiothoracic surgery. **C-RF = C**linical **R**isk **F**actors: congestive heart failure, cerebrovascular disease (stroke, transient ischemic attack); renal insufficiency (creatinine >2); history of myocardial infarction (beyond 30 days), diabetes mellitus. **PFC = P**oor **F**unctional **C**apacity with <4 metabolic equivalents (METS). Patient unable to walk up a flight of steps or walk a level block. **STR** = Refer patient for **S**tress **T**est for ischemic burden evaluation. **2Y-EVAL-NEG** = Within past **2 Ye**a**R**s, if patient has had **EVAL**uation with a stress test showing no inducible ischemia or a normal cardiac catheterization (ie, **NEG**ative) and no change in clinical symptoms or events since the time of last evaluation. **SURG** = Patient may proceed with **SURG**ery

EPIPHANY	PREOP-PT + ACC = E-T PREOP-PT + HRP + C-RF = STR PREOP-PT + HRP + PFC = STR PREOP-PT + C-RF + PFC = STR PREOP-PT + HRP + C-RF + 2Y-EVAL-NEG = SURG PREOP-PT + HRP + PFC = SURG PREOP-PT + C-RF + PFC + 2Y-EVAL-NEG = SURG
DISCUSSION	Preoperative cardiac testing is important to assess for potential perioperative cardiac risk as well assessing the need for postoperative risk stratification and interventions directed at modifying coronary risk factors.
PEARLS	Functional capacity is expressed in metabolic equivalents. 1 MET is defined as 3.5 mL O_2 uptake/kg per min. – Taking care of one's self, such as eating, getting dressed, or using the toilet = 1 MET. – Walking up a flight of steps or one level block = 4 METs. – Doing heavy work around the house such as scrubbing floors or lifting or moving heavy furniture = 4–10 METs. – Participating in strenuous sports such as swimming, singles tennis, football, basketball, and skiing = >10 METs.
REFERENCE	1) Fleisher LA, et al. ACC/AHA 2007 Guidelines on Perioperative Cardiovascular Evaluation and Care for Noncardiac Surgery. *Circulation*. 2007;116:1971–962.

How do I interpret my patients Swanz–Ganz catheterization?

KEY CONCEPT	The interpretation of a Swanz–Ganz catheterization is based upon the measurements of the right atrial pressure, pulmonary artery pressure, pulmonary capillary wedge pressure, and vital signs.
HISTORY	HPI: Dyspnea, palpitations, fatigue, chest pain. PMH: Congestive heart failure, hypertension, pulmonary hypertension, pericarditis. SH: Smoking, alcohol.
PHYSICAL EXAM	Hypotension, fever, peripheral edema, elevated jugular venous pulse, pulsus paradoxus (decrease in systolic blood pressure [>10 mm Hg] on inspiration), Kussmaul's sign (absence of inspiratory decline in jugular venous pressure).
ELECTRO-CARDIOGRAM	Low voltage, sinus tachycardia, electrical alternans (beat to beat QRS variability).
IMAGING	ECHO = Diastolic collapse of right atrium and right ventricle; left atrial collapse; left ventricular ejection fraction <40%; left atrium and ventricular enlargement; wall motion abnormalities. X-ray = Enlarged cardiac silhouette.
SYNTHESIS	**BP** = **B**lood **P**ressure: systolic 120 mm Hg, normal diastolic 80 mm Hg. **RAP** = **R**ight **A**trial **P**ressure: 0–6 mm Hg. **PAP** = **P**ulmonary **A**rtery **P**ressure: systolic 12–30 mm Hg, diastolic 6–12 mm Hg (elevated = PA systolic pressure >35 mm Hg). **PCWP** = **P**ulmonary **C**apillary **W**edge **P**ressure 6–12 mm Hg. **CO** = **C**ardiac **O**utput 5 L/min. **SVR** = **S**ystemic **V**ascular **R**esistance 800–1440 mm Hg. **[I]** = **I**ncreased. **[D]** = **D**ecreased. **CG-SH** = **C**ardio**G**enic **SH**ock. **SS** = **S**eptic **S**hock. **HVL** = **H**ypo**V**o**L**emia. **P-HTN** = **P**ulmonary **H**yper**T**e**N**sion. **TAMP** = **P**ericardial **TAMP**onade

 EPIPHANY	BP[D] + RAP[I] + PAP[I] + PCWP[I] + CO[D] + SVR[I] = CG-SH BP[D] + RA[D] + PAP[D] + PCWP[I] + CO[I] + SVR[D] = SS BP[D] + RA[D] + PAP[D] + PCWP[D] + CO[D] + SVR[I] = HVL PAP[I] = PHTN BP[D] + RA[I] + PA[I] + PCWP[I] + CO[D] + SVR[I] = TAMP
 DISCUSSION	Swanz–Ganz catheterization is an effective and rapid technique for patients in need of hemodynamic monitoring for diagnosis and treatment of shock and complications of heart failure.
 REFERENCE	1) Chatterjee K, et al. The Swan-Ganz Catheters: Past, Present, and Future: A Viewpoint. *Circulation*. 2009;119:147–152.

Does my patient need screening for an abdominal aortic aneurysm (AAA)?

KEY CONCEPT	The goal is to identify patients with AAA before rupture occurs and to balance this against performing an unnecessary test in low risk populations.
HISTORY	HPI: Age, the vast majority of patients will be asymptomatic. PMH: Known vascular disease (coronary artery disease, peripheral vascular disease, collagen vascular disease), risk factors for vascular disease (hypertension, hyperlipidemia, diabetes). FH: Aortic aneurysm or dissection SH: Tobacco use
PHYSICAL EXAM	Pulsatile mass in epigastrium upon palpation.
IMAGING	Abdominal ultrasound: Abdominal aortic diameter >3 cm.
SYNTHESIS	**AAA** = **A**bdominal **A**ortic **A**neurysm **M-60-FAM** = **M**en **60** years of age or older with **FAM**ily history of AAA. **M-65-TOB** = **M**en who are **65** to 75 years of age who have ever used **TOB**acco. **ABD-US** = Refer patient for **ABD**ominal **U**ltra**S**ound for 1-time screening for detection of AAA.
EPIPHANY	**M-60-FAM = ABD-US** **M-65-TOB = ABD-US**

 DISCUSSION	Rupture of an aortic aneurysm is a common cause of death and the mortality of repair is much greater after rupture than elective repair beforehand. There are endovascular and open methods for repair. If a patient is not a candidate for repair should an AAA be discovered, it does not make sense to undertake screening. There are no hard and set rules to screening in many populations due to a lack of data showing it is cost effective. The U.S. Preventive Services Task Force (USPSTF) recommends against the routine screening of women, and the prevalence of AAA is six times lower in women. It is the opinion of the author that screening should be considered in high risk patients who do not fall under the current guidelines based on clinical judgment. Tobacco is the strongest risk factor for AAA.
 PEARLS	– Normal diameter of abdominal aorta is 2 cm. – Ruptured AAA is estimated to cause 5% of sudden deaths and is the 13th most common cause of death.
 REFERENCE	1) Schermerhorn M. A 66-Year-Old Man with an Abdominal Aortic Aneurysm: Review of Screening and Treatment. *JAMA*. 2009;302(18):2015–2022. 2) Hirsch AT. ACC/AHA Guidelines for the Management of PAD. *Circulation*. 2006;113:e463.

ARRHYTHMIAS

How do I manage the rate and rhythm in my patient with atrial fibrillation?

 KEY CONCEPT	Acute management of atrial fibrillation is based on hemodynamic stability and chronic management at preventing symptoms, thromboembolism and heart failure.
 HISTORY	HPI: Duration and severity of symptoms (palpitations, dyspnea, fatigue, lightheadedness, or syncope). Any history of atrial fibrillation and has cardioversion been attempted before. PMH: Hyperthyroidism, hypertension, myocardial infarction, mitral stenosis.
 PHYSICAL EXAM	Irregularly irregular pulse, jugular venous distension, rales, peripheral edema.
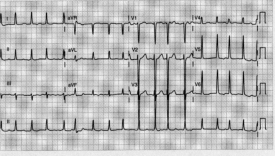 ELECTRO-CARDIOGRAM	Absent P waves, irregularly irregular R-R interval. **Figure 55-1**
 IMAGING	ECHO: Atrial enlargement, left ventricular function, mitral valve function, left atrial appendage velocity, left atrial thrombus.
 SYNTHESIS (cont. on next page)	**AFIB** = **A**trial **FIB**rillation. **RVR** = **R**apid **V**entricular **R**ate: ventricular rate > 100 bpm. **HU** = **H**emodynamically **U**nstable: hypotension (systolic BP < 90 mm Hg) and evidence of shock (mental status changes or decreased urine output). **HS** = **H**emodynamically **S**table: normotensive, normal mentation, no evidence of shock. **SDUR** = Patient with AFIB < 48 hours (**S**hort **DUR**ation). If unknown or doubt as to genuine duration, assume LDUR. **LDUR** = Patient with AFIB > 48 hours (**L**ong **DUR**ation) or unknown duration. **CDV** = Direct current **C**ar**D**io**V**ersion.

 SYNTHESIS (cont. from previous page)	**EL-CDV** = **EL**ective **CDV**: There is time to plan for procedure including informed consent, monitored anesthesia care, and assessing for intracardiac thrombus. If AFIB is LDUR, obtain a transeosopageal echocardiogram prior to CDV. Abort CDV if any thrombus found and reassess after 3 weeks of anticoagulation. **EM-CDV** = **EM**ergent **CDV**: Performed to save the life of the patient at the risk of thromboembolism. **SAE** = **S**earch **A**lternate **E**tiology of shock: Being in AFIB with a normal ventricular rate does not cause shock. **FAIL-CDV** = Patient has had **CDV** in past and reverted back into AFIB. **RC** = **R**ate **C**ontrol with goal of resting HR of 60–80 bpm, and < 110 bpm with mild exertion. For RVR, consider metoprolol 5 mg IV Q15 minutes (max 15 mg) or diltiazem IV bolus 0.25 mg/kg IV followed by 10 mg/hr IV infusion (titrate over the range of 5 to 15 mg/h IV for goal heart rate). For non-acute setting, consider metoprolol PO 25 to 100 mg twice daily or diltiazem 30 to 90 mg 3–4 times daily.
 EPIPHANY	**See chapter on anticoagulation for AFIB in all cases.** **AFIB + RVR + HU = EM-CDV** **AFIB + HU + (NO RVR) = SAE** **AFIB + HS + (NO FAIL-CDV) = RC + EL-CDV** **AFIB + HS + FAIL-CDV = RC**
 DISCUSSION	The primary cause of morbidity and mortality in patients with AFIB is thromboembolism (ex. stroke) that occurs due to stasis of blood in the atria and subsequent thrombus formation that ejects from the heart. Even if a patient reverts back to sinus rhythm, anticoagulation should be continued as AFIB may be paroxysmal and there is still risk for stroke. Rate control is important to prevent cardiac remodeling and the development heart failure (tachycardia-induced cardiomyopathy).
 CONTRA- INDICATIONS	Avoid beta blockers in patients with active reactive airway disease (ex. COPD, asthma). Avoid nondihydropyridine calcium channel blockers (ex. diltiazem) for long term management in patients with left ventricular systolic dysfunction.
 PEARLS	The Atrial Fibrillation Follow-up Investigation of Rhythm Management (AFFIRM) trial showed there was no statistically significant difference in mortality with rate vs. rhythm control.
 REFERENCE	1) Wann LS, et al. 2011 ACCF/AHA/HRS focused update on the management of patients with atrial fibrillation (updating the 2006 guideline). *Circulation.* 2011;123:104–123. 2) Antonielli E, et al. Clinical value of left atrial appendage flow for prediction of long-term sinus rhythm maintenance in patients with nonvalvular atrial fibrillation. *J Am Coll Cardiol.* 2002;39:1443–1449.

Should I start coumadin in my patient with atrial fibrillation?

KEY CONCEPT	The decision to anticoagulate in atrial fibrillation is based on the risk of a thromboembolic event.
HISTORY	HPI: Duration of symptoms (palpitations, dyspnea, fatigue, lightheadedness, or syncope). PMH: Hyperthyroidism, hypertension, heart failure, mitral stenosis, stroke, transient ischemic attack (TIA), any thromboembolism from the heart (ex. to the mesenteric vasculature).
PHYSICAL EXAM	Irregularly irregular pulse, jugular venous distension, rales, peripheral edema.
ELECTRO-CARDIOGRAM	Lack of P waves, irregularly irregular R-R intervals.
IMAGING	ECHO: Atrial enlargement, left ventricular function, mitral valve function, left atrial appendage velocity, left atrial thrombus.
SYNTHESIS	**AFIB** = **A**trial **FIB**rillation. **CHADS2** = Score from 0–6 based on the patient's history: **C** **C**ongestive heart failure [1 point] **H** **H**ypertension [1 point] **A** **A**ge ≥ 75 years [1 point] **D** **D**iabetes mellitus [1 point] **S2** Prior **S**troke or TIA [2 points] **RAS** = **R**isk factors **A**ssociated with **S**troke = Prior stroke, TIA, thromboembolism, or mitral stenosis. **ASA** = Aspirin 325 mg/day (if no contraindications). **AC** = **A**nti**C**oagulation: Must ensure there is no significant contraindication to anticoagulation before initiating. Can use warfarin initiated at 5 mg/day and titrated to target INR of 2.0–3.0. Advantage of warfarin is inexpensive and disadvantage is it requires frequent follow up to adjust dose. Alternate therapy is dabigatran 150 mg twice daily. Advantage is it does not require checking for therapeutic level. Disadvantage is cost and cannot be used with prosthetic valves or significant valve disease, severe renal failure (Creatinine Clearance <15 mL/min) or advanced liver disease.
EPIPHANY	**AFIB + CHADS2 < 2 + (NO RAS) = ASA** **AFIB + CHADS2 < 2 + RAS = AC** **AFIB + CHADS2 ≥ 2 = AC**

DISCUSSION	The primary cause of morbidity and mortality in patients with AFIB is thromboembolism (ex. stroke) that occurs due to stasis of blood in the atria and subsequent thrombus formation that ejects from the heart. Even if a patient reverts back to sinus rhythm, anticoagulation should be continued as AFIB may be paroxysmal and there is still risk for stroke.
PEARLS	The CHADS2 score is directly correlated with risk of stroke: **CHADS2 Score Adjusted Stroke Rate (%/year)** 0 (Low) 1.2–3.0 1–2 (Moderate) 2.8–4.0 3–6 (High) 5.9–18.2
CONTRA-INDICATIONS	In pregnant patients with AFIB, warfarin use should be avoided due to teratogenic effects. Unfractionated heparin during the first trimester and last month of pregnancy can be used as a temporary substitute.
REFERENCE	1) Wann LS, et al. 2011 ACCF/AHA/HRS focused update on the management of patients with atrial fibrillation (updating the 2006 guideline). *Circulation.* 2011;123:104–123. 2) Fang MC, et al. The net clinical benefit of warfarin anticoagulation in atrial fibrillation. *J Am Coll Cardiol.* 2008;51(8):810–815. 3) Gage BF, et al. Selecting patients with atrial fibrillation for anticoagulation:Stroke risk stratification in patients taking aspirin. *Circulation.* 2004;110(16):2287–2292.

How do I manage a patient presenting in acute atrial flutter?

 KEY CONCEPT	The management of acute atrial flutter is based upon reversion to sinus rhythm, maintenance of sinus rhythm, and prevention of systemic embolization.
 HISTORY	HPI: Palpitations, lightheadedness, dyspnea, syncope. PMH: Congestive heart failure, myocardial infarction, rheumatic heart disease, hyperthyroidism, pericarditis. PSH: Coronary artery bypass graft.
 ELECTRO-CARDIOGRAM	P waves absent, biphasic "sawtooth" flutter waves present at a rate of about 300 beats/min, ventricular rate >150 beats/min, narrow QRS complex.
 IMAGING	ECHO = Left atrial thrombus, left atrial size.
 SYNTHESIS	**AFLUT** = Patient diagnosed **A**trial **FLUT**ter on ECG of less than 48-hour duration. **HS** = **H**emodynamically **S**table: patient not hypotensive, in cardiogenic shock, or displaying mental status changes. **HUSL** = **H**emodynamically **U**n**S**tab**L**e: patient with hypotension, cardiogenic shock, mental status changes. **P-REV** = **P**harmacological **REV**ersion with ibutilide (0.1 mg/kg over 10 minutes if patient <60 kg or 1 mg over 10 minutes if patient >60 kg; if patient fails to revert to sinus rhythm, repeat dose again). **RC** = **R**ate **C**ontrol with goal of resting HR of 80 bpm and 110 bpm with moderate exercise. Administer metoprolol 5 mg IV Q5 minutes (max 15 mg) or digoxin 0.25 mg IV Q2 hours (max 1.5 mg) in patients with heart failure and no accessory pathway. **CDV** = Refer patient for direct current **C**ar**D**io**V**ersion. **CHADS2** = See chapter "Should I start anticoagulation in my patient with AFIB?" **CATH-ABL** = Refer patient for radio-frequency catheter ablation to prevent recurrence of atrial flutter. **AC** = **O**ral **A**nti**C**oagulation with warfarin. Target INR of 2–3 and in patients with mechanical heart valves a target INR of 2.5–3.5. **ASA** = **A**spirin 325 mg/day orally.
E **EPIPHANY**	**Controlling rate:** **AFLUT + HS = RC + P-REV** **AFLUT + HUSL = CDV** **Anticoagulation:** **AFLUT + CHADS2 >= 2 = AC** **AFLUT + CHADS2 <2 = ASA**

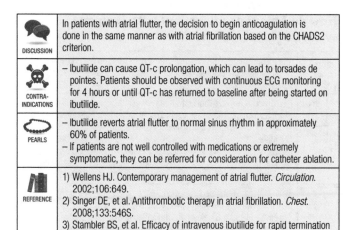

DISCUSSION	In patients with atrial flutter, the decision to begin anticoagulation is done in the same manner as with atrial fibrillation based on the CHADS2 criterion.
CONTRA-INDICATIONS	– Ibutilide can cause QT-c prolongation, which can lead to torsades de pointes. Patients should be observed with continuous ECG monitoring for 4 hours or until QT-c has returned to baseline after being started on ibutilide.
PEARLS	– Ibutilide reverts atrial flutter to normal sinus rhythm in approximately 60% of patients. – If patients are not well controlled with medications or extremely symptomatic, they can be referred for consideration for catheter ablation.
REFERENCE	1) Wellens HJ. Contemporary management of atrial flutter. *Circulation*. 2002;106:649. 2) Singer DE, et al. Antithrombotic therapy in atrial fibrillation. *Chest*. 2008;133:546S. 3) Stambler BS, et al. Efficacy of intravenous ibutilide for rapid termination of atrial flutter. *Circulation*. 1996;94:1613–1621.

How do I manage my patient with Brugada syndrome?

KEY CONCEPT	The management of Brugada syndrome is focused on the prevention of sudden cardiac death (SCD) and balancing that against unnecessary invasive therapies.
HISTORY	HPI: Syncope, exercise capacity. PMH: Sudden cardiac arrest, ventricular tachycardia, syncope. FH: Brugada syndrome, unexplained sudden death SH: Male MED: Cardiac sodium channel blocker [procainamide], calcium channel blocker [diltiazem], beta blocker [propanolol], tricyclic antidepressants [amitryptiline], selective serotonin reuptake inhibitor [fluoxetine].
ELECTRO-CARDIOGRAM	Type I: Coved ST-segment elevation >=2 mm (0.2 mV) at J-point with negative T wave in >=2 right precordial leads (V1–V3). Type II: Saddleback ST-elevation with a high takeoff ST elevation >=2 mm, a trough displaying >=1 mm ST elevation, and either a positive or biphasic T wave. Type III: Saddleback or coved ST-segment elevation of <1 mm. Right bundle branch block (RBBB) or incomplete RBBB.
SYNTHESIS	**BRUG** = Patient diagnosed with **BRUG**ada syndrome type I, II or III on ECG. **HRISK** = Patient is High **RISK** for sudden cardiac death: Patient has had an episode of sudden cardiac death, documented malignant arrhythmia (ventricular tachycardia or ventricular fibrillation), or a strong clinical suspicion of having serious arrhythmias (syncope). **PREF** = Patient **PREF**erence to have ICD: After careful discussion of risks versus benefits and taking into account special circumstances (such as a strong family history of sudden death), patients may opt for ICD as primary prevention. **MED-TX** = Medical therapy: Start Quinidine bisulfate 300 mg po q6h to prevent deterioration into malignant arrhythmias. **ICD** = Refer patient for placement of **I**mplantable **C**ardioverter-**D**efibrillator.
E EPIPHANY	**BRUG = MED-TX** **BRUG + HRISK = ICD** **BRUG + PREF = ICD**
DISCUSSION	In patients with Brugada syndrome who are at high risk, an ICD placement is preferred over quinidine because it is more effective in preventing sudden cardiac death.

  CONTRA-INDICATIONS	– Quinidine can prolong QT-c interval, which can lead to torsades de pointes, and should be monitored upon initiation of treatment.
  PEARLS	– Patients with Brugada syndrome and a history of syncope have a 2.5 times higher risk of sudden cardiac death than patients with no history of syncope.
  REFERENCE	1) Belhassen B, et al. Efficacy of quinidine in high-risk patients with Brugada syndrome. *Circulation.* 2004;110:1731–1737. 2) Epstein AE, et al. ACC/AHA/HRS 2008 guidelines for device-based therapy of cardiac rhythm abnormalities. *Circulation.* 2008;117:e350.

How do I manage 3rd degree atrioventricular block?

KEY CONCEPT	The management of 3rd degree atrioventricular (AV) block is based upon the identification and treatment of reversible causes first, and placement of pacemaker if indicated
HISTORY	HPI: Assess presence and severity of symptoms: syncope, lightheadedness, dyspnea, palpitations. PMH: CAD, congestive heart failure, hypertension, hypersensitive carotid sinus syndrome. FH: AV block PSH: Catheter ablation. MED: Calcium channel blockers, beta blockers, digitalis, amiodarone, adenosine, quinidine, procainamide.
ELECTRO-CARDIOGRAM	PR interval irregularly variable, no association (dissociation) between P wave and QRS.
SYNTHESIS	**3-AVB** = Patient diagnosed with **3**rd degree **A**trio**V**entricular **B**lock on ECG. **BC** = Significant bradycardia: ventricular rate < 55 bpm or periods of asystole > 3 seconds. **HU** = **H**emodynamically **U**nstable: hypotension (systolic BP < 90 mm Hg) and evidence of shock (mental status changes or decreased urine output). **HS** = **H**emodynamically **S**table: normotensive, normal mentation, no evidence of shock. **TPM** = Temporary pacemaker: Placed emergently. May use transcutaneous pacing pads or transvenous pacemaker. **T-REV** = **T**reat **REV**ersible cause of 3-AVB: – Stop medications that impair AV conduction (ex: calcium channel blockers, beta-blockers, digitalis, amiodarone, adenosine, quinidine, procainamide). – Correct electrolytes (esp. K, Ca, and Phos). – Evaluate and treat myocardial ischemia (see this chapter) – Reduce increased vagal tone (eg, treat abdominal pain). **PPM** = Permanent pacemaker. Placed electively after 3-AVB persists after reversible causes are treated. Patient referred to electrophysiology for placement.
E **EPIPHANY**	**3-AVB + BC + HU = TPM + T-REV + PPM** **3-AVB + BC + HS = T-REV + PPM**

DISCUSSION	In patients where reversible causes of 3rd degree AV block have been ruled out, pacemaker placement will reestablish conduction from the sinoatrial node to the AV node.
PEARLS	The basic approach to a patient with 3-AVB is: 1) stabilize (may require temporary pacing), 2) identify and treat reversible causes, and 3) evaluate for permanent pacing.
REFERENCE	1) Epstein AE, et al. ACC/AHA/HRS 2008 guidelines for device-based therapy of cardiac rhythm abnormalities. *Circulation.* 2008;117:e350.

How do I manage my patient with 2nd degree type I (Wenckebach) atrioventricular block?

KEY CONCEPT	The management of 2nd degree type 1 (Wenckebach) atrioventricular (AV) block is based upon the identification and treatment of reversible causes and placement of pacemaker if indicated.
HISTORY	HPI: Syncope, angina, heart failure. PMH: CAD, congestive heart failure, hypertension, hypersensitive carotid sinus syndrome. FH: AV block. MED: Calcium channel blockers, beta blockers, digitalis, amiodarone, adenosine, quinidine, procainamide.
ELECTRO-CARDIOGRAM	Progressive PR interval prolongation followed by a nonconducted P wave.
SYNTHESIS	**2-AVB-1** = Patient diagnosed with **2**nd degree **AV** Block type **1** on ECG. **REV** = **REV**ersible cause of 2-AVB-1 such as increased vagal tone (carotid massage producing asystole >3 seconds), myocardial ischemia (stress echocardiogram), or drugs (calcium channel blockers, beta blockers, digitalis, amiodarone, adenosine, quinidine, procainamide) that suppress atrioventricular conduction. **T-REV** = If present, **T**reat **REV**ersible cause of 2-AVB-1. – Increased vagal tone refer for pacemaker placement. – Myocardial ischemia, see chapter on positive stress test. – Discontinue medication (calcium channel blockers, beta blockers, digitalis, amiodarone, adenosine, quinidine, procainamide) causing impaired AV conduction. **PM** = Refer patient for **P**ace**M**aker placement. **SBC** = **S**ymptomatic **B**rady**C**ardia: heart rate <55 bpm with syncope, lightheadedness, fatigue, or exercise intolerance. **ASYS-3** = Period of **ASYS**tole lasting >3 seconds or escape rate <40 bpm. **EXER** = 2-AVB-1 occurring during **EXER**cise in absence of myocardial ischemia. **V-40** = **V**entricular rate >**40** bpm with left ventricular dysfunction, cardiomegaly, or block below the AV node. **POST-MI** = 2-AVB-1 occurring following **M**yocardial **I**nfarction. **NMD** = **N**euro**M**uscular **D**iseases such as myotonic muscular dystrophy, or peroneal muscular atrophy. **ABL** = 2-AVB-1 occurring after catheter ablation of AV-junction.

EPIPHANY	**2-AVB-1 + REV = T-REV** **2-AVB-1 + SBC = PM** **2-AVB-1 + ASYS-3 = PM** **2-AVB-1 + EXER = PM** **2-AVB-1 + V-40 = PM** **2-AVB-1 + POST-MI = PM** **2-AVB-1 + NMD = PM** **2-AVB-1 + ABL = PM**
DISCUSSION	In patients with 2nd degree AV block reversible causes should be evaluated before pacemaker placement is considered.
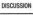 **PEARLS**	– The distinction between type I and type II 2nd degree AV block cannot be made when there is a 2:1 block (every other beat is dropped) as there is no way to observe the PR prolongation.
REFERENCE	1) Epstein AE, et al. ACC/AHA/HRS 2008 guidelines for device-based therapy of cardiac rhythm abnormalities. *Circulation.* 2008;117:e350.

How do I manage my patient with 2nd degree type II atrioventricular block?

KEY CONCEPT	The management of 2nd degree type II atrioventricular (AV) block is based upon the identification and treatment of reversible causes and placement of pacemaker if indicated.
HISTORY	HPI: Syncope, angina, heart failure. PMH: CAD, congestive heart failure, hypertension, hypersensitive carotid sinus syndrome. FH: AV block. MED: Calcium channel blockers, beta blockers, digitalis, amiodarone, adenosine, quinidine, procainamide.
ELECTRO-CARDIOGRAM	Prolonged PR interval of fixed duration followed by a P wave that fails to conduct to the ventricles, wide QRS complex.
SYNTHESIS	**2-AVB-2** = Patient diagnosed with **2**nd degree **AV B**lock type 1 on ECG. **REV** = **REV**ersible cause of 2-AVB-2 such as increased vagal tone (carotid massage producing asystole >3 seconds), myocardial ischemia (stress echocardiogram), or drugs (calcium channel blockers, beta blockers, digitalis, amiodarone, adenosine, quinidine, procainamide) that suppress atrioventricular conduction. **T-REV** = If present, **T**reat **REV**ersible cause of 2-AVB-2. – Increased vagal tone, refer for pacemaker placement. – Myocardial ischemia, see chapter on positive stress test. – Discontinue medication (calcium channel blockers, beta blockers, digitalis, amiodarone, adenosine, quinidine, procainamide) causing impaired AV conduction. **PM** = Refer patient for **Pa**ce**M**aker placement. **SBC** = **S**ymptomatic **B**rady**C**ardia: heart rate <55 bpm with syncope, lightheadedness, fatigue, or exercise intolerance. **ASYS-3** = Period of **ASYS**tole lasting >**3** seconds or escape rate <40 bpm. **EXER** = 2-AVB-2 occurring during **EXER**cise in absence of myocardial ischemia. **V-40** = **V**entricular rate >**40** bpm with left ventricular dysfunction, cardiomegaly, or block below the AV node. **POST-MI** = 2-AVB-2 occurring following **M**yocardial **I**nfarction. **NMD** = **N**euro**M**uscular **D**iseases such as myotonic muscular dystrophy or peroneal muscular atrophy. **ABL** = 2-AVB-2 occurring after catheter ablation of AV junction.

EPIPHANY	2-AVB-2 + REV = T-REV 2-AVB-2 + SBC = PM 2-AVB-2 + ASYS-3 = PM 2-AVB-2 + EXER = PM 2-AVB-2 + V-40 = PM 2-AVB-2 + POST-MI = PM 2-AVB-2 + NMD = PM 2-AVB-2 + ABL = PM
DISCUSSION	In patients with 2nd degree AV block, reversible causes should be evaluated before pacemaker placement is considered.
PEARLS	– AV block can be provoked by exercise and is most often due to disease in the His–Purkinje system.
REFERENCE	1) Epstein AE, et al. ACC/AHA/HRS 2008 guidelines for device-based therapy of cardiac rhythm abnormalities. *Circulation*. 2008;117:e350.

Is it ok for my patient to consume an energy beverage?

KEY CONCEPT	The decision to permit one's patient to consume an energy beverage is based upon medical condition and level of physical activity and fitness.
HISTORY	PMH: Coronary artery disease (CAD), hypertension, congestive heart failure (CHF), arrhythmias (heart block, supraventricular tachycardia, atrial fibrillation). SH: Alcohol.
ELECTRO-CARDIOGRAM	Q waves, heart block.
IMAGING	ECHO: LVEF <40%, LA and LV enlargement, wall motion abnormalities.
SYNTHESIS	**EB** = **E**nergy **B**everage containing greater than 140 mg of caffeine per 16 ounces. **ATH** = **ATH**lete = exercising most days of the year and involved in competitive athletic activities. **N-ATH** = **N-ATH**lete = not exercising most days of the year and not involved in competitive athletic activities. **1-CAN-EB** = Limit consumption of EB to <500 mL or **1 CAN**/day. Do not mix **EB** with alcohol. Rehydrate with water after intense physical activity or exercise. Consult health professional if experience any side effects to EB. **AVOID** = **AVOID** consumption of EB. **MED-COND** = Patient with following **MED**ical **COND**itions: hypertension, CAD, CHF, or history of arrhythmias. **CONS** = **CONS**ult physician before using EB.
EPIPHANY	**ATH = AVOID** **N-ATH = 1-CAN-EB** **N-ATH + MED-COND = CONS**
DISCUSSION	Ingestion of an energy beverage before intense physical activity can have serious adverse effects such as restlessness, irritability, dehydration, and increased blood pressure. Individuals with underlying heart disease should consult with their physicians before consumption of an energy beverage.

PEARLS

– Adverse effects of caffeine typically manifest with ingestion higher than 200 mg; these include insomnia, nervousness, headache, tachycardia, arrhythmia, and nausea.

REFERENCE

1) Higgins JP, et al. Energy beverages: content and safety. *Mayo Clin Proc.* 2010;85(11):1033–1041.

Does this ECG show changes of hyperkalemia?

KEY CONCEPT	In patients with hyperkalemia (potassium >5 mEq/L), changes will manifest on ECG as well as the patient may manifest signs and symptoms.
HISTORY	HPI: Muscle weakness beginning in legs and progressing to arms, paralysis. PMH: Renal tubular acidosis, hypoaldosteronism, renal failure, diabetes. LABS: Potassium >5 mEq/L.
ELECTRO-CARDIOGRAM	ECG: Tall-peaked T waves, shortened QT interval, progressive lengthening of PR interval and QRS duration.
SYNTHESIS	**ECG-HYPERK = ECG** changes with **HYPERK**alemia seen are tall-peaked T waves, shortened QT interval, progressive lengthening of the PR interval and QRS duration. **SUS-HYPERK = SUS**pect **HYPERK**alemia based on ECG findings alone. **LAB-HYPERK** = K >5 mEq/L. **HYPERK** = Confirmed diagnosis of **HYPERK**alemia.
E **EPIPHANY**	**ECG-HYPERK = SUS-HYPERK** **SUS-HYPERK + LAB-HYPERK = HYPERK**
DISCUSSION	Marked ECG changes and physical manifestations of hyperkalemia usually occur when serum potassium concentration is ≥7.0 mEq/L or at lower levels with an acute rise in serum potassium.
PEARLS	– Hyperkalemia can lead to sinus bradycardia, sinus arrest, slow idioventricular rhythm, ventricular tachycardia, ventricular fibrillation, asystole.
REFERENCE	1) Wagner GS. *Marriotts Practical Electrocardiography*. 10th ed. New York, NY: Lippincott Williams and Wilkins; 2000. 2) Mattu A, et al. Electrocardiographic manifestations of hyperkalemia. *Am J Emerg Med.* 2000 Oct;18(6):721–729.

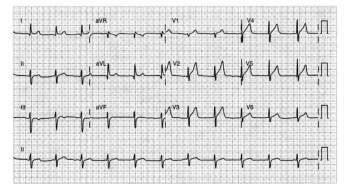

Figure 63–1

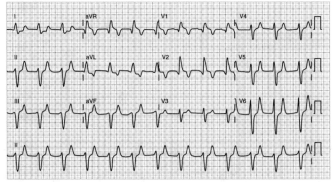

Figure 63–2

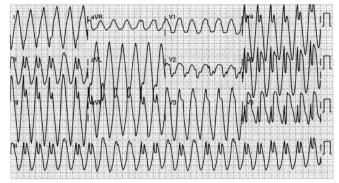

Figure 63–3

Does this ECG show changes of hypokalemia?

KEY CONCEPT	In patients with hypokalemia [potassium < 3.5 mEq/L] changes may manifest on the electrocardiogram.
HISTORY	HPI: Muscle weakness (classicly beginning in legs and progressing to arms), paralysis, tetany, dyspnea, nausea/vomiting. PMH: Diarrhea, Conn's syndrome, hypomagnesemia. MED: Loop diuretic [ex. furosemide], thiazide diuretic [ex. hydrochlorothiazide] LABS: Potassium < 3 mEq/L
ELECTRO-CARDIOGRAM	ECG: Depression of ST segment, decreased amplitude of T wave, U waves in V4-V6. Figure 64–1
SYNTHESIS	**E-STD** = **E**CG shows **ST**-segement **D**epression **E-DAMPTW** = **E**CG shows **D**ecreased **AMP**litute of **T** **W**ave **E-UW** = ECG shows **U** **W**ave (seen best in V4-V6) **SUS-HYPOK** = **SUS**pect **HYPOK**alemia based on ECG findings alone. If seen, obtain serum potassium level unless ECG abnormalities are unchanged from prior ECG and potassium level was normal at that time. **LAB-HYPOK** = plasma potassium (**K**) < 3.5 mEq/L. **HYPOK** = confirmed diagnosis of **HYPOK**alemia.
EPIPHANY	**E-STD + E-DAMPTW + E-UW = SUS-HYPOK** **LAB-HYPOK = HYPOK**

DISCUSSION	Marked ECG changes and physical manifestations of hypokalemia usually occur when serum potassium concentration is <2.5 mEq/L (defined as severe hypokalemia).
PEARLS	– Hypokalemia can lead to rhabdomyolysis as potassium release from muscle cells normally mediates vasodilation and increased blood flow to muscles during exercise; decreased potassium leads to a decreased blood flow to muscles during exercise.
REFERENCE	1) Wagner GS. *Marriotts Practical Electrocardiography*. 10th ed. New York, NY: Lippincott Williams and Wilkins; 2000. 2) Shintani S, et al. Marked hypokalemic rhabdomyolysis with myoglobinuria due to diuretic treatment. *Eur Neurol.* 1991;31(6):396–398.

Does this ECG show changes of hypercalcemia?

KEY CONCEPT	In patients with hypercalcemia (calcium >11 mEq/L), changes will manifest on ECG as well as physically.
HISTORY	HPI: Constipation, muscle weakness, fatigue, confusion, polyuria, polydypsia, dehydration, nausea. PMH: Hyperparathyroidism, malignancy, chronic kidney disease, nephrolithiasis. LABS: Calcium >11 mEq/L.
ELECTRO-CARDIOGRAM	ECG: Shortened QT interval, PR prolongation, upstroke of initial portion of T wave, increased amplitude of QRS, biphasic T waves.
SYNTHESIS	**ECG-HIGH-CA** = **ECG** changes with **HIGH CA**lcium seen are shortened QT interval, PR prolongation, upstroke of initial portion of T-wave, increased amplitude of QRS, biphasic T waves. **HYPER-C** = **HYPER**calcemia. **LAB-HI-CA** = **LAB** showing **HI**gh **CA**lcium level (>11 mEq/L).
EPIPHANY	**ECG-HIGH-CA + LAB-HI-CA = HYPER-C**
DISCUSSION	Patients with serum calcium levels <12 mg/dL may be asymptomatic but may exhibit symptoms such as fatigue or constipation. A serum calcium level of 12–14 mg/dL will most often manifest with symptoms of muscle weakness, polyuria, nausea, dehydration, and/or polydypsia.

PEARLS	– Chronic hypercalcemia may lead to deposition of calcium in heart valves, coronary arteries, and myocardium, resulting in hypertension and cardiomyopathy.
REFERENCE	1) Wagner GS. *Marriotts Practical Electrocardiography*. 10th ed. New York, NY: Lippincott Williams and Wilkins; 2000.

Does this ECG show changes of hypocalcemia?

KEY CONCEPT	In patients with hypocalcemia (calcium <9 mg/dL), changes will manifest on ECG, as well as the patient may manifest signs and symptoms.
HISTORY	HPI: Tetany, seizure, anxiety. PMH: Hypoparathyroidism, vitamin D deficiency or resistance, chronic renal failure. PSH: Head and neck surgery (thyroidectomy). LABS: Calcium <9 mg/dL.
PHYSICAL EXAM	Trousseau sign (carpopedal spasm by inflation of a sphygmomanometer above systolic blood pressure for three minutes), Chvostek sign (contraction of facial muscles elicited by tapping the facial nerve anterior to ear), papilledema.
ELECTRO-CARDIOGRAM	ECG: Prolonged QT interval (>0.45 seconds in males and >0.47 seconds in females).
SYNTHESIS	**ECG-HYPOCA** = **ECG** changes seen with low calcium or **HYPOCA**lcemia are prolonged QT interval (>0.45 seconds in males and >0.47 seconds in females). **SUS-HYPOCA** = **SUS**pect **HYPOCA**lcemia based on ECG findings alone. **LAB-HYPOCA** = **LAB** showing **HYPOCA**lcemia, ie, calcium <9 mg/dL. **HYPOCA** = Confirmed diagnosis of **HYPOCA**lcemia.
EPIPHANY	**ECG-HYPOCA = SUS-HYPOCA** **SUS-HYPOCA + LAB-HYPOCA = HYPOCA**
DISCUSSION	Acute hypocalcemia is characterized by neuromuscular irritability or tetany, which can manifest as perioral numbness, paresthesias of the hands and feet, muscle cramps, or severe carpopedal spasm, laryngospasm.

PEARLS	– Torsades de pointes can be triggered by hypocalcemia due to prolongation of QT interval.
REFERENCE	1) Wagner GS. *Marriotts Practical Electrocardiography*. 10th ed. New York, NY: Lippincott Williams and Wilkins; 2000.

Does this ECG show right bundle branch block?

KEY CONCEPT	In patients with right bundle branch block (RBBB), changes will manifest on ECG.
HISTORY	HPI: Dyspnea, cough, chest pain. PMH: Right ventricular hypertrophy, cor pulmonale, hypertension, coronary artery disease. PSH: Right heart catheter insertion.
ELECTRO-CARDIOGRAM	ECG: QRS duration >0.12 seconds, qRS or qrS in lead I and V6, ST depression and T-wave inversion in right precordial leads (V1–V3), ST-T vectors are discordant to terminal mean QRS spatial vector. **Figure 67–1**
SYNTHESIS	**ECG-RB** = QRS duration >0.12 seconds, qRS or qrS in lead I and V6, ST depression and T wave inversion in right precordial leads (V1–V3), ST-T vectors are discordant to terminal mean QRS spatial vector. **RBBB** = **R**ight **B**undle **B**ranch **B**lock.
EPIPHANY	**ECG-RB = RBBB**

DISCUSSION	Right bundle branch block is a common finding on ECG, which increases in prevalence with age.
PEARLS	– The left anterior descending artery is the major blood supply of the right bundle branch.
REFERENCE	1) Wagner GS. *Marriotts Practical Electrocardiography*. 10th ed. New York, NY: Lippincott Williams and Wilkins; 2000.

Does this ECG show left bundle branch block?

KEY CONCEPT	In patients with left bundle branch block (LBBB) changes will manifest on the electrocardiogram.
HISTORY	HPI: May be asymptomatic, chest pain, dyspnea, palpitations. PMH: Coronary artery disease, hypertension, heart failure, myocardial infarction.
ELECTRO-CARDIOGRAM	ECG: QRS >0.12 seconds; loss of Q wave and wide slurred R wave in lead I, aVL, and v6; rS or QS in V1; ST depression and T wave inversion in V4–v6; ST elevation and upright T waves in right precordial leads (V1–V3). Figure 68–1
SYNTHESIS	**WIDE-QRS** = **QRS** >0.12 sec; **R-CHANGE** = Loss of Q wave and wide slurred R wave in lead I, aVL, and v6; rS or QS in V1; **ST-CHANGE** = **ST** depression and **T** wave inversion in V4–v6; ST elevation and upright T waves in right precordial leads [V1–V3]. **LBBB** = **L**eft **B**undle **B**ranch **B**lock.
EPIPHANY	**WIDE-QRS + R-CHANGE + ST-CHANGE = LBBB**

DISCUSSION	Left bundle branch block most commonly occurs in individuals with underlying heart disease and/or worsening heart disease and left ventricular function.
PEARLS	– Left ventricular hypertrophy is commonly present alongside LBBB; however, it is difficult to diagnose ECG as LBBB produces similar changes. It is usually established by echocardiography.
REFERENCE	1) Wagner GS. *Marriotts Practical Electrocardiography*. 10th ed. New York, NY: Lippincott Williams and Wilkins; 2000.

Does this ECG show left ventricular hypertrophy?

KEY CONCEPT	In patients with left ventricular hypertrophy (LVH) changes will manifest on ECG.
HISTORY	HPI: May be asymptomatic, dyspnea on exertion, chest pain PMH: Hypertension, heart failure, coronary artery disease, aortic stenosis.
ELECTRO-CARDIOGRAM	ECG: Left axis deviation; sum of S wave in V1 and R wave in V5 or V6 is >35 mm; R wave in aVL is >11 mm. S in V3 plus R in aVL is >28 mm in men; S in V3 + R in aVL is 20 mm in women. Figure 69–1
SYNTHESIS	**ECG-LV** = Left axis deviation; **VOLT1** = **VOLT**age criteria #**1**: Sum of S wave in V1 and R wave in V5 or V6 is >35 mm; **VOLT2** = **VOLT**age criteria #**2**: R wave in aVL is >11 mm. **VOLT3** = **VOLT**age criteria #**3**: S in V3 plus R in aVL is >28 mm (men) or >20 mm (women). **LVH** = **L**eft **V**entricular **H**ypertrophy.
EPIPHANY	**ECG-LV + VOLT1 = LVH** **ECG-LV + VOLT2 = LVH** **ECG-LV + VOLT3 = LVH**

DISCUSSION	The increase in QRS voltage seen in left ventricular hypertrophy is due to the increase in myocardial muscle fibers.
PEARLS	– LVH increases the risk of heart failure, ventricular arrhythmias, death following myocardial infarction, and a cerebrovascular event.
REFERENCE	1) Wagner GS. *Marriotts Practical Electrocardiography*. 10th ed. New York, NY: Lippincott Williams and Wilkins; 2000.

Does this ECG show second degree type I atrioventricular block?

◖—◯ KEY CONCEPT	In patients with second degree type I [Wenckebach] atrioventricular (AV) block, changes will manifest on the electrocardiogram.
HISTORY	HPI: Syncope, angina, heart failure. PMH: CAD, congestive heart failure, hypertension, hypersensitive carotid sinus syndrome. FH: AV block.
ELECTRO-CARDIOGRAM	ECG: A general look at the ECG will often show a pattern of "grouped beating." Progressive PR interval prolongation followed by a nonconducted P wave. **Figure 70–1**
SYNTHESIS	**E-PVAR** = PR interval is variable and gradually increases from beat to beat, resets after a dropped beat. **E-PFAIL** = ECG shows discernable P waves that fail to conduct to the ventricles (no QRS complaex tied to that P wave). **2-AVB-1** = **2**nd degree **A**trio**V**entricular **B**lock Type **1**.
E EPIPHANY	**E-PVAR + E-PFAIL = 2-AVB-1**

 DISCUSSION	Patients with second degree type I (Wenckebach) AV block typically have a benign course and can be followed up in the outpatient setting.
 PEARLS	– The distinction between type I and type II 2nd degree AV block cannot be made when there is a 2:1 block (every other beat is dropped), as there is no way to observe the PR prolongation.
 REFERENCE	1) Wagner GS. *Marriotts Practical Electrocardiography*. 10th ed. New York, NY: Lippincott Williams and Wilkins; 2000. 2) Epstein AE, et al. ACC/AHA/HRS 2008 guidelines for device-based therapy of cardiac rhythm abnormalities. *Circulation*. 2008;117:e350.

Does this ECG show second degree type II atrioventricular block (Mobitz II)?

KEY CONCEPT	In patients with second degree type II atrioventricular (AV) block, changes will manifest on electrocardiogram.
HISTORY	HPI: Syncope, angina, heart failure. PMH: CAD, congestive heart failure, hypertension, hypersensitive carotid sinus syndrome. FH: AV block.
ELECTRO-CARDIOGRAM	ECG: A general look at the ECG will often show a pattern of "grouped beating." Prolonged PR interval of fixed duration followed by a P wave which fails to conduct to the ventricles, narrow QRS complex. **Figure 71–1**
SYNTHESIS	**E-PFIX** = ECG shows a fixed PR interval. **E-PFAIL** = ECG shows discernable P waves that fail to conduct to the ventricles (no QRS complaex tied to that P wave). **2-AVB-2** = Second degree **A**trio**V**entricular **B**lock Type **2**.
EPIPHANY	**E-PFIX + E-PFAIL = 2-AVB-2**
DISCUSSION	Second degree type II AV block commonly involves the AV node and can progress to complete heart block if untreated.

PEARLS

– AV block can be provoked by exercise and is most often due to disease in the His–Purkinje system.

REFERENCE

1) Wagner GS. *Marriotts Practical Electrocardiography*. 10th ed. New York, NY: Lippincott Williams and Wilkins; 2000.
2) Epstein AE, et al. ACC/AHA/HRS 2008 Guidelines for Device-Based Therapy of Cardiac Rhythm Abnormalities. *Circulation*. 2008;117:e350.

Does this ECG show third degree atrioventricular block?

KEY CONCEPT	In patients with third degree atrioventricular (AV) block, changes will manifest on electrocardiogram.
HISTORY	HPI: Syncope, dizziness, dyspnea, palpitations. PMH: CAD, congestive heart failure, hypertension, hypersensitive carotid sinus syndrome. FH: AV block PSH: Catheter ablation.
ELECTRO-CARDIOGRAM	ECG: PR interval irregularly variable, dissociation between P wave and QRS, wide QRS complex. Figure 72–1
SYNTHESIS	**E-PVAR** = PR interval is variable. **E-DIS** = No association (dissociation) between P waves and QRS complexes. The atrial rate (P-P interval) is often different than the ventricular rate (R-R interval). The QRS duration may be wide if there is a ventricular escape rhythm. **3-AVB** = **3**rd degree **A**trio**V**entricular **B**lock.
EPIPHANY	**E-PVAR + E-DIS = 3-AVB**
DISCUSSION	Third degree AV block occurs when there is complete failure of the AV node to conduct any impulses from the atria to the ventricles. Typically a ventricular escape rhythm is present with a widened QRS complex.

|
PEARLS | – Third degree AV block occurring below the level of the bundle of His is typically associated with a narrow QRS complex. |
|
REFERENCE | 1) Wagner GS. *Marriotts Practical Electrocardiography.* 10th ed. New York, NY: Lippincott Williams and Wilkins; 2000. |

What should I do if my patient has premature ventricular contractions?

KEY CONCEPT	The management of premature ventricular contractions (PVC) is based on the presence or absence of symptoms.
HISTORY	HPI: Chest pain, palpitations, fatigue, dizziness, syncope, hyperventilation; asymptomatic with ECG findings of PVC. PMH: Hypertension, mitral valve prolapse, coronary artery disease, hypertrophic/dilated cardiomyopathy, heart failure. SH: Caffeine, alcohol, smoking.
ELECTRO-CARDIOGRAM	QRS duration >120 msec, bizarre QRS morphology, T wave in the opposite direction from the main QRS vector, fully compensatory pause. Figure 73–1
SYNTHESIS	**PVC** = **P**remature **V**entricular **C**ontraction present on ECG. **SYMP** = **SYMP**tomatic patient experiencing chest pain, fatigue, syncope, hyperventilation. **ASYMP** = **ASYMP**tomatic patient. **OBS** = **OBS**erve patient for development of symptoms. **PROP** = **PROP**anolol 1 mg/dose every 2 minutes, maximum 5 mg. **AMIO** = **AMIO**darone 800 mg/day for 1 week.
EPIPHANY	**PVC + ASYMP = OBS** **PVC + SYMP = PROP + AMIO**
DISCUSSION	PVC's occur in a broad spectrum of the population and are commonly diagnosed during auscultation or routine ECG's.

 CONTRA- INDICATIONS	**Do not begin AMIO if:** – Cardiogenic shock. – Severe sinus-node dysfunction causing marked sinus bradycardia. – Second or third degree atrioventricular block. – Episodes of bradycardia that have caused syncope (except when used in conjunction with a pacemaker).
 PEARLS	– Hypertension increases the prevalence of PVCs by 23%.
 REFERENCE	1) Zipes DP, et al. ACC/AHA/ESC 2006 Guidelines for Management of Patients With Ventricular Arrhythmias and the Prevention of Sudden Cardiac Death—Executive Summary. *JACC.* 2006;48(5):1064–1108. 2) Simpson RJ Jr. Prevalance of premature ventricular contractions in a population of African American and white men and women; the atherosclerosis risk in communities (ARIC). *Am Heart J.* 2002;143:535–540.

How do I manage a patient who presents with WPW?

 KEY CONCEPT	Ventricular pre-excitation from an accessory pathway (bundle of Kent) causing abnormal communication from atria to ventricles leading to unstable arrhythmias.
 HISTORY	Most individuals are asymptomatic but also present with palpitations, dizziness, shortness of breath, and syncope. A few patients can present with sudden cardiac arrest/death.
 PHYSICAL EXAM	Tachycardia.
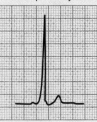 ELECTRO-CARDIOGRAM	Delta wave (slurred upstroke of QRS). Short PR interval and slightly widened QRS. Positive r wave in V1 if pathway is between RA/RV, negative delta wave in V1 if pathway is between LA/LV. Wide complex tachycardia if atrial fibrillation is present. **Figure 74–1**
 IMAGING	Echocardiogram: Evaluate for underlying heart disease (Epstein anomaly).
 SYNTHESIS (cont. on next page)	**Evaluation** **DE** = If **D**elta wave disappears with **E**xercise. **DER** = If **D**elta wave present during **R**est and **E**xercise. **O** = **O**bserve. **EP** = **EP** consult for programed electrical stimulation **Acute treatment** **U** = **U**nstable: if patient is tachycardic, hypotensive, altered mental status, and overall unstable. **DC** = **DC** Cardioversion. **NCT** = Patient has **N**arrow **C**omplex **T**achycardia. **AFRVR** = If patient has **A**trial **F**ibrillation with **R**apid **V**entricular **R**esponse.

 SYNTHESIS (cont. from previous page)	**TM** = **T**erminating **M**aneuvers: first attempt valsalva/carotid massage, then if unsuccessful try adenosine/verapamil (5 mg q2 minutes up to 15 mg) or possible DC cardioversion if refractory. **ANT** = **ANT**iarrhythmics: amiodarone or procainamide. <div align="center">**Chronic**</div>**SYM** = If patient has episodes of **SYM**ptomatic tachycardias, has high risk occupation (pilot, athlete), concurrent atrial fibrillation. **RFA** = **R**adiofrequency **A**blation. **ASMY** = If patient is asymptomatic and <35 years. **ASMO** = If patient is asymptomatic and >35 years. **EPS** = **EPS** testing and risk stratification.
 EPIPHANY	<div align="center">**Evaluation:**</div>**DE = 0** **DER = EP** <div align="center">**Acute treatment:**</div>**U = DC** **NCT = TM** **AFRVR = ANT** <div align="center">**Chronic treatment:**</div>**SYM = RFA** **ASMY = EPS** **ASMO = 0**
 DISCUSSION	Most patients with WPW who do not experience tachycardia do not need treatment and can be observed. Treatment is indicated when patients are symptomatic and/or unstable. Most patients may never develop symptoms, and conduction via the accessory pathway disappears as the patient grows older. The ECG can vary depending upon other factors that can alter the frequency of impulses conducted across the accessory pathway (stress, adrenaline states, diet: caffeine). Radiofrequency ablation is the treatment of choice and is often curative.
 PEARLS	Avoid adenosine and all AV nodal blockers (BB, CCB, digoxin) if patient has atrial fibrillation or atrial flutter. This combination of atrial fibrillation and WPW is considered dangerous, and most antiarrhythmic drugs are contraindicated.
 REFERENCE	1) Rosner MH, Brady WJ Jr, Kefer MP, Martin ML. Electrocardiography in the patient with the Wolff–Parkinson–White syndrome: diagnostic and initial therapeutic issues. *Am J Emerg Med.* 1999;17(7):705–714 2) Mehta D, Wafa S. Relative efficacy of various physical maneuvers in the termination of junctional tachycardia. *Lancet* 1988;1:1181 3) Belardinelli L, Linden J. The cardiac effects of adenosine. *Prog Cardiovasc Dis.* 1989;32:73

How do I acutely manage a patient with torsade de pointes (TdP)?

KEY CONCEPT	Torsade de pointes (TdP) is a form of ventricular tachycardia with differing QRS morphology (polymorphic) and can be rapidly fatal.
HISTORY	HPI: Syncope, angina, dyspnea, unresponsive PMHx: Long-QT syndrome, heart failure, presence of defibrillator Meds: QT prlonging drugs (See QTc chapter)
PHYSICAL EXAM	Unresponsive, hypotension, tachycardia, diaphoresis
ELECTRO-CARDIOGRAM	Rapid polymorphic ventricular tachycardia. Prolonged QT. Rotation of electrical axis. Long and short RR intervals. Figures 75–1 and 75–2
IMAGING	CXR/Echo to rule out structural abnormalities.

 SYNTHESIS	**TdP** = **T**orsade **d**e **P**ointes is present on ECG or telemetry right now. **TERM-TdP** = **TERM**inated **T**orsade **d**e **P**ointes. May be self terminated or successful cardioversion. **RECUR-TdP** = **R**ecurrent **TdP**. **HU** = **H**emodynamically **U**nstable: hypotension (systolic BP < 90 mm Hg) and evidence of shock (mental status changes or decreased urine output). **HS** = **H**emodynamically **S**table: normotensive, normal mentation, no evidence of shock. **EM-CDV** = **EM**ergent **CDV**: Performed to save the life of the patient. **INC-HR** = **INC**rease **H**eart **R**ate. A faster heart rate decreases the QT interval and decreases the chance of TdP recurrenc. Can use isoproterenol 5 mcg/min or overdrive electrical pacing. **MED-TX** = **MED**ical **T**reatment: Telemetry monitoring, replete electrolytes (especially magnesium and potassium, would give at least 2 gm magnesium sulfate empirically), stop QT prolonging drugs, rule out myocardial ischemia. **EP** = **E**lectro**P**hysiology consultation. Patient should be evaluated for defibrillator placement and may need further evaluation for long-QT syndrome. **ARTIFACT** = Occasionally motion of ECG leads will appear to be TdP such as when a patient is brushing teeth. Careful examination of the strips will reveal QRS complexes hidden in the artifact. If a patient is awake, talking, and pleasant, a careful review should be done to evaluate for artifact.
 EPIPHANY	**TdP + HU = EM-CDV** **TERM-TdP + HS = MED-TX + EP** **RECUR-TdP = INC-HR + MED-TX + EP** **ARTIFACT = Reassurance**
 DISCUSSION	Torsades is associated with long QT syndrome that has characteristic PVC (R on T) phenomenon on ECG. It can be an inherited ion channel mutation or drug toxicity/electrolyte abnormality that affects conduction across certain ion channels. Long-term management may include (1) ICD placement if avoiding offending agent does not work; (2) pacemaker if patient has bradycardia or AV block; (3) beta blockers (propranolol, esmolol, nadolol); and (4) sympathectomy.
 PEARLS	TdP can be rapidly fatal and is an acute emergency. The main treatment of TdP occurring right now is electric cardioversion. TdP is strongly linked to long QT syndrome. See QTc chapter for QT prolonging drugs.
 REFERENCE	1) Drew BJ, et al. Prevention of Torsade de Pointes in Hospital Settings. *Circulation*. 2010;121:1047–1060. 2) Hoshino K, et al. Optimal administration dosage of magnesium sulfate for torsades de pointes in children with long QT syndrome. *J Am Coll Nutr*. 2004;23(5):497S–500S.

Does this ECG show Wolff–Parkinson–White syndrome?

KEY CONCEPT	In patients with Wolff–Parkinson–White syndrome, changes will manifest on ECG.
HISTORY	HPI: Asymptomatic or symptoms of palpitations, dizziness, dyspnea, syncope. PMH: Long QT syndrome, atrial fibrillation.
ELECTRO-CARDIOGRAM	ECG: PR interval <0.12 seconds; QRS >0.12 seconds; delta wave (slurred upstroke of QRS). **Figure 76–1**
SYNTHESIS	**ECG-WPW** = PR interval <0.12 seconds; QRS >0.12 seconds; delta wave (slurred upstroke of QRS). **WPW** = **W**olff–**P**arkinson–**W**hite syndrome.
EPIPHANY	**ECG-WPW = WPW**
DISCUSSION	Patients can also present with atrial fibrillation and extremely rapid ventricular response (>200 bpm) due to ability of bypass tract to pre-excite the ventricles.

 PEARLS	– Wolff–Parkinson–White syndrome is seen in 0.2% of the general population.
 REFERENCE	1) Wagner GS. *Marriotts Practical Electrocardiography*. 10th ed. New York, NY: Lippincott Williams and Wilkins; 2000. 2) Koplan BA, et al. ACC/AHA 2007 guidelines on perioperative cardiovascular evaluation and care for noncardiac surgery. *Circulation*. 2010;122:e480–e483.

Does this ECG show atrioventricular nodal reentry tachycardia?

⊷O **KEY CONCEPT**	In patients with atrioventricular nodal reentry tachycardia (AVNRT), changes will manifest on electrocardiogram.
HISTORY	HPI: Palpitations, dizziness, dyspnea, chest pain. FH: AV nodal reentry tachycardia.
ELECTRO-CARDIOGRAM (cont. on next page)	ECG: Ventricular rate between 120–220 beats/min; narrow QRS (<0.12 seconds); P wave buried with or fused with QRS complex. Figure 77–1 Figure 77–2

 ELECTRO-CARDIOGRAM (cont. from previous page)	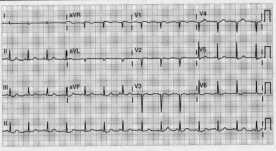 **Figure 77–3**
 SYNTHESIS	**E-VR** = **E**CG shows **V**entricular **R**ate between 120–220 beats/min. **E-QRS** = **E**CG shows narrow **QRS** [< 0.12 sec]. **E-P** = **E**CG shows **P** wave buried in or fused with QRS complex. **AVNRT** = **A**trio**V**entricular **N**odal **R**eentry **T**achycardia.
E EPIPHANY	**E-VR + E-QRS + E-P = AVNRT**
 DISCUSSION	In AVNRT the slow pathway conducts first from the atria to the ventricles, resulting in a long P-R interval, followed by the fast pathway conducting back up to the atria resulting in a short R-P interval.
 PEARLS	– AVNRT occurs in approximately 10% of the general population and accounts for up to two-thirds of all cases of paroxysmal supraventricular tachycardia.
 REFERENCE	1) Wagner GS. *Marriotts Practical Electrocardiography*. 10th ed. New York, NY: Lippincott Williams and Wilkins; 2000. 2) Denes P, et al. Dual atrioventricular nodal pathways — A common electrophysiological response. *Br Heart J.* 1975;37:1069–1076.

Does this ECG show arrhythmogenic right ventricular dysplasia?

KEY CONCEPT	In patients with arrhythmogenic right ventricular dysplasia (ARVD), changes will manifest on ECG.
HISTORY	HPI: Palpitations, syncope, chest pain, dyspnea. PMH: syncope, history of sudden cardiac deaths, palpitations, tachycardia FH: sudden cardiac death, prior genetic testing
ELECTRO-CARDIOGRAM	ECG: QRS prolongation >110 msec in V1; prolongation of S-wave upstroke; Epsilon wave (distinct wave between end of QRS and onset of T wave); inverted T waves in right precordial leads (V1–V3).
SYNTHESIS	**AVRD** = **A**rrhythmogenic **R**ight **V**entricular **D**ysplasia. **ECG-AVRD** = QRS prolongation > 110msec in V1; prolongation of S-wave upstroke; Epsilon wave (distinct wave between end of QRS and onset of T wave); inverted T waves in right precordial leads (V1–V3).
E **EPIPHANY**	**ECG-AVRD = AVRD**
DISCUSSION	ARVC is characterized by a macroscopically fatty appearance of the right ventricular free wall, which produces regional wall motion and conduction abnormalities. The diagnosis can be confirmed by doing further imaging studies including echocardiography, cardiac computed tomography, or cardiac magnetic resonance.

|
PEARLS | – ECG is normal in 40–50% of patients upon initial presentation. |
|
REFERENCE | 1) Marcus FI, et al. Diagnosis of arrhythmogenic right ventricular cardiomyopathy/dysplasia. *Circulation.* 2010;121:1533.
2) Jaoude SA, et al. Progressive ECG changes in arrhythmogenic right ventricular dysplasia. *Eur Heart J.* 1996;17(11):1717–1722. |

Does this ECG show a prolonged QT interval?

○—○ KEY CONCEPT	On ECG the QT interval can be measured and calculated to account for changes in heart rate based upon the RR interval.
HISTORY	HPI: Palpitations, syncope, seizures, and/or cardiac arrest. PMH: Congenital long QT syndrome (LQTS), bradycardia, atrial fibrillation, congestive heart failure. MED: Amiodarone, digitalis (see chapter on drugs that prolong QT interval).
ELECTRO-CARDIOGRAM	ECG: QT-c is the QT interval that is corrected for heart rate. QT-c = QT interval/(square root of RR interval). Prolonged QT-c interval is >0.44 seconds. Figure 79–1
SYNTHESIS	**ECG-QT** = QT-c >0.45 seconds in males and >0.47 seconds in females. **PROL-QT** = **PROL**onged **QT** interval.
EPIPHANY	**PROL-QT = ECG-QT**
DISCUSSION	Patients at risk for prolonged QT interval should be monitored as it can develop into torsade de pointes.

PEARLS	1) QT-c >0.5 seconds is high risk for torsade de pointes.
REFERENCE	1) Wagner GS. *Marriotts Practical Electrocardiography.* 10th ed. New York, NY: Lippincott Williams and Wilkins; 2000.

Does this ECG show tricyclic antidepressant toxicity?

KEY CONCEPT	In patients with tricyclic antidepressant (TCA), toxicity changes will manifest on ECG.
HISTORY	HPI: Patient taking TCA (amitryptiline, imipramine, nortriptyline) with confusion, delirium, palpitations, hypotension, hyperthermia. PMH: Depression, post-traumatic stress disorder, attention-deficit hyperactivity disorder, anxiety disorder.
ELECTRO-CARDIOGRAM	ECG: Prolongation of QRS >100 msec, deep slurred S waves in leads I and avL, R wave in AVR >3 mm, R-to-S ratio in AVR >0.7
SYNTHESIS	**ECG-TCA** = **ECG** changes seen in **TCA** toxicity are prolongation of QRS >100 msec; deep slurred S waves in leads I and aVL; R wave in AVR >3 mm; R-to-S ratio in AVR >0.7. **TCA-TOX** = **TCA TOX**icity.
EPIPHANY	**ECG-TCA = TCA-TOX**
DISCUSSION	In patients presenting with symptoms of TCA toxicity, an ECG should be obtained as a life-threatening arrhythmia can develop quickly.

| PEARLS | – Prolongation of QRS of >100 msec had a 26% of developing a seizure and those with a QRS >160 msec had a 50% chance of developing a ventricular arrhythmia. |
| REFERENCE | 1) Wagner GS. *Marriotts Practical Electrocardiography*. 10th ed. New York, NY: Lippincott Williams and Wilkins; 2000. |

In this young healthy patient, is this an abnormal ECG or normal variant, and what should I do next?

 KEY CONCEPT	Certain abnormal ECG findings are seen as normal variants in young healthy athletes.
 HISTORY	HPI: Young symptomatic healthy adult who presents with findings on routine ECG.
 IMAGING	ECG: Review old tracings to exclude new significant disease.
SYNTHESIS (cont. on next page)	Identify the ECG patterns that can be mistaken as abnormal. **RSA = R**espiratory **S**inus **A**rrhythmia: change in R-R interval from respiration shortened during inspiration and prolonged during expiration, physiologic to match ventilation and perfusion. **VAGO** = Pronounced **VAGO**tonia in athletes: sinus bradycardia, first degree AV blocks, supraventricular and ventricular ectopic beats. These do not require attention if they are asymptomatic or do not produce pauses greater than 4 seconds. Ectopic beats are no more frequent in athletes than the general population. **BER = B**enign **E**arly **R**epolarization: isolated J point elevation. ST/T ratio is <0.25 and normalizes with isoproteronol or exercise (used to distinguish from pericarditis). **IRBBB = I**ncomplete **R**ight **B**undle **B**ranch **B**locks: QRS <0.12 seconds, seen in patients with skeletal abnormalities. **PJTW = P**ersistent **J**uvenile **T**-**W**ave pattern: T-wave inversion in V1-3, but upright in other leads. The T vector is oriented left and posterior from heart orientation in chest. Seen also in potassium deficiency, vagotonia, hyperventilation. **PHT = P**hysiologic **H**yper**T**rophy: adaptation from static or dynamic exercise. Common variants are increased voltage, prominent U waves, intraventricular conduction delays, early repolarization, increased QT intervals. **PROM-T = PROM**inent **T**-wave amplitude: T waves tall but not symmetric, seen in vagotonia, hyperkalemia, anemia. **STD = ST** segment **D**epression: seen in excess sympathetic activity, hyperventilation, neurocirculatory asthenia. **QW = Q W**aves: seen in vertical or horizontal heart/chest abnormalities/ elderly. Lack of multiple leads with Q waves differentiates normal variants with old infarctions. **PRWP = P**oor **R**-**W**ave **P**rogression: differentiate old anterior MI with the presence of Q waves. **ASYM = ASYM**ptomatic patient. **SYM = SYM**ptomatic patient: patient who reports significant symptoms (especially with exercise), including chest pain, dyspnea, presyncope/ syncope, or palpitations.

 SYNTHESIS (cont. from previous page)	**REASS** = **REASS**ure patient and tell them they likely have a normal variation on their ECG, and they should be fine; if they develop any symptoms, return for reevaluation. **ECHO** = Order an **ECHO**cardiogram to rule out significant structural heart disease. **STR-ECHO** = Order a **STR**ess **ECHO**cardiogram to rule out structural as well as functional problems that might be leading to their symptoms.
E EPIPHANY	**ASYM + RSA/VAGO/BER/IRBBB/PJTW/PRWP = REASS** **ASYM + PHT/PROM-T/QW/PRWP = ECHO** **ASYM + STD = STR-ECHO** **SYM = STR-ECHO**
 DISCUSSION	Knowing the normal ECG variant is important to screen against patients that may be mistaken for underlying silent cardiovascular disorders and prevent unnecessary workup/evaluation. Abnormal ECG in young individuals may represent underlying silent cardiomyopathy such as HOCM, dilated cardiomyopathy, long QT syndrome, and arrhythmogenic right ventricular cardiomyopathy. However, many conditions are benign and are seen as physiologic adaptations from exercise. Misinterpretation of the normal variants leads to wrong diagnosis and treatment. When in doubt, careful interpretation of resting ECG recordings and review of old tracings are recommended to exclude significant disease.
 PEARLS	Exercise reversible ST elevation and T-wave changes are physiologic changes. Simple arrhythmias usually disappear with exercise. Deep inspiration, valsalva, potassium administration, or propranolol may normalize juvenile T waves. Physiologic hypertrophy has normal systolic and diastolic function. Exercise-induced sudden cardiac death in athletes is unusual without preexisting heart disease. The prevalence of HOCM in trained athletes is rare; such changes associated with HOCM select out individuals from sports. If significant ST depression is seen in ECG, ischemia should be excluded. It may be difficult to differentiate a healthy athlete with athletic heart from an athletic patient with a diseased heart by resting ECG, if LVH criteria are met echocardiography and exclusion of ischemia is recommended. Complex ventricular forms of arrhythmia should be evaluated for cardiomyopathy. Athletes with benign early repolarization with chest pain need to differentiate with pericarditis, myocarditis, ST-elevation infarction. AV block or Mobitz 2nd/3rd blocks are unusual and are a sign of organic lesion until proved otherwise. Arrhythmias that become more frequent or symptomatic during exercise ECG warrant more testing.
 REFERENCE	1) Higgins JP. Normal resting electrocardiographic variants in young athletes. *Phys Sportsmed.* 2008;36(1):1–7.

Sinus arrhythmia

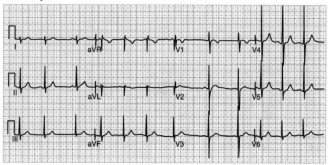

Figure 81–1

Benign repolarization

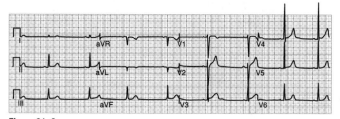

Figure 81–2

Athlete heart

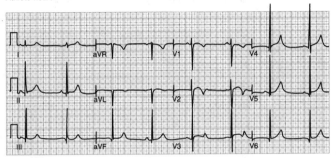

Figure 81–3

Poor R wave progression

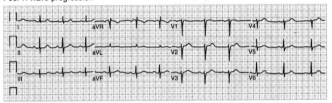

Figure 81–4

How do I manage a patient with right bundle branch block?

KEY CONCEPT	Defect in right-side electrical conduction system where the right heart is depolarized via the left bundle. The right ventricle is thus depolarized later than the left.
HISTORY	HPI: Patient presents with right bundle branch block PMH: palpitations, dizziness, syncope, history of congenital heart disease PSH: cardiac surgery FH: heart block, arrhythmias, pacemakers, sudden cardiac death, infarctions
PHYSICAL EXAM	Wide and persistently splitting S2 with respiratory variation.
ELECTRO-CARDIOGRAM	QRS >100 msec. Terminal R wave in V1 (rR′, rsR′, qR, R). Slurred S wave in I, V6. There should be terminal QRS and T-wave discordance.
IMAGING	Echocardiogram: Evaluate for increased RV pressure (cor pulmonale), RVH.
SYNTHESIS	**RBBB** = **R**ight **B**undle **B**ranch **B**lock on ECG. **TWD** = **T**-**W**ave **D**iscordance = the T wave is deflected in the direction opposite the terminal deflection of the QRS complex. **TWC** = **T**-**W**ave **C**oncordance = the T wave is in the same direction as the terminal deflection of the QRS complex. **CS-STE** = **C**oved or **S**addleback **ST**-segment **E**levation: coved ST-segment elevation $>=2$ mm (0.2 mV) at J-point with negative T wave in $>=2$ right precordial leads (V1–V3) or saddleback ST-segment elevation with a high takeoff ST-segment elevation of $>=2$ mm, a trough displaying $>=1$ mm ST elevation, and either a positive or biphasic T wave or saddleback or coved ST-segment elevation of <1 mm—consider. **SYNC** = **SYNC**ope. **REASS** = **REASS**ure, and no further workup required at this time. **ISCH** = Perform **ISCH**emic burden evaluation (eg, stress test). **BRUG** = Consider **BRUG**ada syndrome and refer for further evaluation (eg, electrophysiology evaluation). **PPM** = Refer for consideration of **P**ermanent **P**ace**M**aker placement.
EPIPHANY	**RBBB + TWD = REASS** **RBBB + TWC = ISCH.** **RBBB + CS-STE = BRUG** **RBBB + SYNC = PPM**

DISCUSSION	A right bundle branch block does not cause harm in otherwise healthy people. The prevalence increases with age, and there is no association for ischemia, infarction, or death.
	Pathologic etiologies include hypertension, cardiomyopathy, congenital heart disease, myocarditis fibrosis of the conduction system (Lenegre disease), and interventions.
PEARLS	Concordant terminal QRS and T wave may suggest ischemia or infarction.
REFERENCE	1) Rotman M, Triebwasser JH. A clinical and follow-up study of right and left bundle branch block. *Circulation.* 1975;51:477

CONGENITAL HEART DISEASES

Does a patient with an atrial septal defect require closure?

 KEY CONCEPT	The decision to close an atrial septal defect (ASD) is based upon the size and degree of shunting.
 HISTORY	HPI: May be asymptomatic. Dyspnea, exercise intolerance, palpitations. PMH: Arrhythmias, pulmonary hypertension, congestive heart failure (CHF) FH: Family History of congenital heart disease
 PHYSICAL EXAM	May have a normal examination. Prominent right ventricular (RV) impulse, wide fixed splitting of S2, midsystolic pulmonary ejection murmur.
 ELECTRO-CARDIOGRAM	Prolonged PR interval. Secundum ASD = Right axis deviation + right atrial enlargement + incomplete right bundle branch block (IRBBB). Primum ASD = Left axis deviation + IRBBB.
 IMAGING	Chest X-ray: RV and RA enlargement; prominent pulmonary artery; increased pulmonary vascularity. Echocardiogram: Direct visualization of ASD or shunting (especially with agitated saline study), dilation of the right atrium/ventricle, elevated pulmonary pressure, Qp/Qs (pulmonary to systemic ratio) to quantitate shunt.
SYNTHESIS	**SYM** = **SYM**ptomatic ASD = Dyspnea on exertion, fatigue, palpitations, evidence of atrial arrhythmias. **ASYM** = **ASYM**ptomatic ASD **SIG-SHUNT** = Significant left to right shunt (usually caught on echo), Qp:Qs > 1.5. **STR-CHANGE** = Evidence of **STR**uctural **CHANGE**s in the heart such as elevated pulmonary pressure, right atrial or right ventricular enlargement or hypertrophy. **PxE** = History of a paradoxical embolic event. **CLOSURE** = **CLOSURE** of ASD. Can be performed percutaneously or surgically depending on size and location of ASD. **FOLLOW** = Clinical follow up and echocardiogram every 2 years or sooner if symptoms develop. **END-STAGE** = The clinical picture from an uncorrected significant ASD over time. May have severe irreversible pulmonary hypertension or Eisenmenger's physiology. Mortality is not improved with closure at this point. Prognosis is poor. **MED-TX** = Medical management. There is no medicine to correct the anatomical defect. Can give medicines to alleviate right heart failure and pulmonary hypertension.

EPIPHANY	**SYM + (NO END-STAGE) = CLOSURE** **ASYM + SIG-SHUNT = CLOSURE** **ASYM + STR-CHANGE = CLOSURE** **ASYM + PxE = CLOSURE** **ASYM + (NO SIG-SHUNT) + (NO STR-CHANGE) = FOLLOW** **END-STAGE = MED-TX**
DISCUSSION	Most patients with ASD are asymptomatic for decades and have a relatively normal physical exam making ASD the most common adult uncorrected congenital anomaly. The natural history for an ASD with a significant shunt is to develop pulmonary hypertension and right heart remodeling from pulmonary vascular overload. The mortality once severe pulmonary hypertension has developed is high. Closure of ASD has a very low incidence of morbidity and mortality from the procedure itself and can be done percutaneously or surgically. The goal is to close significant ASDs early before complications develop. Very small ASDs without significant shunting rarely become clinically significant.
CONTRA-INDICATIONS	– Closure is not recommended in patients with severe irreversible pulmonary artery hypertension.
PEARLS	– Most patients with ASD will be asymptomatic for decades. – Mortality is increased with significant shunts due to pulmonary vascular overload, and can be improved with closure even when patients are older or asymptomatic. – Once severe irreversible pulmonary hypertension has developed outcomes are not improved with closure. – Small ASDs with trivial shunts usually are not clinically significant.
REFERENCE	1) Warnes CA, Williams RG, Bashore TM, et. al. ACC/AHA 2008 Guidelines for Adults with CHD. *J Am Coll Cardiol.* 2008 Dec 2;52(23):e174–e176. 2) Brickner ME, et al. Congenital Heart Disease in Adults—First of Two Parts. *N Engl J Med.* 2000;342(4):256–263. 3) Du ZD, et al. Comparison Between Transcatheter and Surgical Closure of Secundum Atrial Septal Defect in Children and Adults: Results of a Multicenter Nonrandomized Trial. *J Am Coll Cardiol.* 2002;39(11):1836–1844.

How do I manage my patient with a patent foramen ovale?

KEY CONCEPT	The management of a patient with a patent foramen ovale (PFO) is based upon the risk of developing a cryptogenic stroke.
HISTORY	HPI: Syncope, paralysis, dyspnea, cyanosis, or migraine headache. PMH: Thromboembolic event, cerebrovascular accident, hypercoagulable state (factor V Leiden, antithrombin deficiency, protein C and S deficiency), transient ischemic attack (TIA).
IMAGING	ECHO: Presence of right to left shunt across the interatrial septum with agitated saline contrast study.
SYNTHESIS	**PFO** = Patient with documented **P**atent **F**oramen **O**vale. **TIA** = Patient with **T**ransient **I**schemic **A**ttack. **CRST** = Patient with prior **CR**yptogenic **ST**roke (stroke occurring in the absence of an identified cardioembolic or large vessel source and with a distribution that is not consistent with small vessel disease). **HCS** = **H**yper**C**oagulable **S**tate (factor V Leiden, antithrombin deficiency, protein C and S deficiency) or history of venous thromboembolism (deep venous thrombosis). **RCS** = Patient with **R**ecurrent **C**ryptogenic **S**troke despite medical therapy. **ASP** = **ASP**irin 325 mg/day. **AC** = Oral **A**nti**C**oagulation with warfarin, target INR of 2–3. **CLOS** = Refer patient for **CLOS**ure of PFO.
E EPIPHANY	**PFO + TIA = ASA** **PFO + CRST = ASA** **PFO + HCS = AC** **PFO + RCS = CLOS**
DISCUSSION	Patients with a PFO are at an increased risk for the development of a cryptogenic stroke. Anticoagulation with warfarin is recommended in patients with a hypercoagulable state or history of venous thrombosis, as studies have shown the benefits outweigh the risks when compared to aspirin.
PEARLS	– PFO occurs in 25% of the general population. – In patients <55 years with cryptogenic stroke, 46% were found to have a PFO. – Patients with a larger size PFO have a higher recurrence rate of cryptogenic stroke.

REFERENCE

1) Sacco RL, et al. Guidelines for Prevention of Stroke in Patients with Ischemic Stroke or Transient Ischemic Attack. *Circulation*. 2006;113:e409–e449.
2) Hidehiko H, et al. Patent Foramen Ovale: Current Pathology, Pathophysiology, and Clinical Status. *J Am Coll Cardiol*. 2005;46:1768–1776.

Should I refer my patient with an isolated ventricular septal defect for closure?

KEY CONCEPT	The decision to refer a patient for closure of a ventricular septal defect (VSD) is based upon left ventricular function, degree of left to right shunting, pulmonary artery pressure, and presence of endocarditis.
HISTORY	HPI: Systolic murmur, dyspnea, orthopnea, or cyanosis. PMH: Congestive heart failure, pulmonary artery hypertension.
PHYSICAL EXAM	Holosystolic murmur at left lower sternal border.
ELECTRO-CARDIOGRAM	Biventricular hypertrophy or isolated right ventricular hypertrophy.
IMAGING	ECHO: Size and location of defect, number of defects, calculation of QP/QS, presence of left to right shunt, ventricular size and function. X-ray: Left atrial and left ventricular enlargement, increased pulmonary vascular markings.
SYNTHESIS	**VSD** = Patient with documented **V**entricular **S**eptal **D**efect. **CLOSURE** = Refer patient for surgical **CLOSURE** of VSD. **QPQS** = Pulmonary to systolic blood flow ratio (QP/QS) measured by echocardiogram or cardiac catheterization (normally in the absence of shunts, the flow through both pulmonary and system circulation should be the same so the **QP/QS** ratio should be 1.0). **LVOVD** = Clinical evidence of **L**eft **V**entricular volume **OV**erloa**D** (usually noted as diastolic interventricular septal flattening resulting in a "D" shaped left ventricle on echocardiogram during diastolic relaxation). **IE** = Patient with history of **I**nfective **E**ndocarditis. **L-R-S** = **L**eft to **R**ight **S**hunting across VSD. **PAP** = **P**ulmonary **A**rtery **P**ressure less than two-thirds of systemic pressure. **PVR** = **P**ulmonary **V**ascular **R**esistance less than two-thirds of systemic vascular resistance **LVF** = **L**eft **V**entricular systolic or diastolic **F**ailure.
EPIPHANY	VSD + QPQS >2.0 + LVOVD = CLOSURE VSD + IE = CLOSURE VSD + L-R-S + QPQS >1.5 + PAP + PVR = CLOSURE VSD + L-R-S + QPQS >1.5 + PVR = CLOSURE VSD + L-R-S + QPQS >1.5 + LVF = CLOSURE

DISCUSSION	Patients with VSD and elevated QP/QS, abnormal left ventricular function, or history of IE should be referred for surgical closure to prevent the development of pulmonary hypertension or Eisenmenger's syndrome.
CONTRA-INDICATIONS	– VSD closure is not recommended in patients with severe irreversible pulmonary artery hypertension.
PEARLS	– VSD is the most common congenital heart defect at birth. – Seventy percent of VSDs are located in the membranous portion of the interventricular septum, with the majority of these closing spontaneously by the age of 12.
REFERENCE	1) Warnes CA, et al. ACC/AHA 2008 Guidelines for the Management of Adults with Congenital Heart Disease. *J Am Coll Cardiol.* 2008;52:e174–e176. 2) Brickner ME. Congenital Heart Disease in Adults. *NEJM.* 2000;342:256–263.

HEART FAILURE AND HYPERTENSION

How do I manage systolic heart failure?

KEY CONCEPT	The management of systolic heart failure is based upon relieving symptoms of volume overload [congestion, dyspnea] and improving left ventricular function.
HISTORY	HPI: Dyspnea on exertion or at rest, fatigue, weakness, diaphoresis. PMH: Hypertension, coronary artery disease, hyperlipidemia, diabetes, atrial fibrillation.: PSH: Smoking, alcohol.
PHYSICAL EXAM	Peripheral edema, elevated jugular venous pressure, rales, laterally displaced apical impulse, S3 gallop.
IMAGING	ECHO: LVEF <40%, LA and LV enlargement, wall motion abnormalities. X-ray: Cardiomegaly, cephalization of pulmonary vessels [increased distribution of flow to apices], pleural effusion.
SYNTHESIS	**S-HF** = Patient with **S**ystolic **H**eart **F**ailure, LVEF <40%. **LVEF** = **L**eft **V**entricular **E**jection **F**raction. **AFIB** = **A**trial **FIB**rillation. **FUROS** = **FUROS**emide 40 mg IV load followed by 20 mg/hr. **ACEI** = **ACE**-Inhibitor enalapril 10 mg BID. If patient unable to tolerate ACE inhibitors, give angiotensin II receptor blocker (ARB) valsartan orally 80 mg BID. **METO** = Oral extended release **METO**prolol 25 mg QD. **DIG** = **DIG**oxin 0.5 mg QD for 2 days followed by 0.25 QD maintenance dose. **HYD** = **HYD**ralazine 10 mg TID. **NIT** = Isosorbide di**NIT**rate 20 mg TID. **INTOL-ACEI** = Patients who are **INTOL**erable to **ACE I**nhibitors or angiotensin II receptor blockers. **INEFF** = **INEFF**ective treatment with furosemide and enalapril, with patient exhibiting symptoms of heart failure (dyspnea, weakness, elevated BP).
E **EPIPHANY**	**S-HF = FUROS + ACEI + METO** **S-HF + INTOL-ACEI = FUROS + HYD + NIT + METO** **S-HF + INEFF = FUROS + ACEI (or HYD+NIT) + METO + DIG** **S-HF + AFIB = FUROS + ACEI + METO + DIG** **S-HF + AFIB + INTOL-ACEI = FUROS + HYD + NIT + METO + DIG**

DISCUSSION	Digoxin is effective in increasing cardiac output, improving exercise capacity and left ventricular function in patients with systolic heart failure unresponsive to diuretics, ACE inhibitors, and beta blockers. While neurohormonal effects occur with doses of digoxin < 0.25 mg/day, positive inotropic actions usually require doses >= 0.25 mg/day.
PEARLS	– DIG trial has shown digoxin therapy to significantly reduce hospitalization rates for patients with heart failure, but no benefits in overall mortality.
REFERENCE	1) Hunt SA, et al. 2009 Focused update incorporated into the ACC/AHA 2005 guidelines for the diagnosis and management of heart failure in adults. *Circulation*. 2009;119:e391. 2) Digitalis Investigation Group. Sex based differences in the effect of digoxin for the treatment of heart failure. *N Engl J Med*. 1997;336:525–533.

How do I manage a patient presenting with acute diastolic heart failure?

KEY CONCEPT	Diastolic heart failure (DHF) is defined as heart failure (HF) with a preserved LVEF variably defined as LVEF >45% or 50%. The management of diastolic heart failure is based upon reducing congestive state, controlling heart rate, treatment and prevention of ischemia, and control of blood pressure.
HISTORY	HPI: Dyspnea on exertion or at rest, fatigue, weakness, diaphoresis. PMH: Hypertension, coronary artery disease, hyperlipidemia, diabetes, atrial fibrillation. SH: Smoking, alcohol.
PHYSICAL EXAM	Peripheral edema, elevated jugular venous pressure, rales, laterally displaced apical impulse, S3 gallop, irregularly irregular pulse.
IMAGING	ECHO: LVEF >50%, diminished early diastolic filling, increased late diastolic filling.
SYNTHESIS	**ADHF** = **A**cute **D**iastolic **H**eart **F**ailure. **AFIB** = **A**trial **FIB**rillation present. **REST-SR** = **REST**ore **S**inus **R**hythm in patient. **SR** = **S**alt **R**estriction <2 g/day. **FUROS** = Diuretic **FUROS**emide: recommended in all patients with clinical symptoms of volume overload: FUROSemide 40 mg IV load followed by 40 mg IV every 12 hours or 20 mg/hr IV infusion. **ACEI** = **A**ngiotensin **C**onverting **E**nzyme **I**nhibitor (ACEI): recommended in patients with diastolic HF with symptomatic atherosclerotic disease and/or diabetes. If systolic blood pressure >90 mm Hg give enalapril 10 mg orally BID or lisinopril 5 mg orally QD. If patient unable to tolerate ACE inhibitors, give angiotensin II receptor blocker (ARB) valsartan orally 80 mg BID. Do not give if renal function significantly abnormal (serum Cr >2.0 mg/dL). **BB** = **B**eta **B**locker: recommended in patients with diastolic HF and prior MI, hypertension, and/or atrial fibrillation: metoprolol 50 mg orally every 6 hours or atenolol 20 mg orally QD (do not give to patient with PR interval >0.24 seconds, 2nd or 3rd degree heart block, active asthma or reactive airways disease). **ISCH** = Patient exhibiting symptoms of **ISCH**emia (chest pain, tightness/discomfort). **NIT** = Isosorbide di**NIT**rate 20 mg orally TID. **EVAL** = **EVAL**uate patient for acute coronary syndrome, see chapter on UA/NSTEMI management. **HCTZ** = **H**ydro**C**hloro**T**hia**Z**ide 25 mg orally QD.

 EPIPHANY	**ADHF = SR + FUROS + ACEI + BB** **ADHF + ISCH = SR + FUROS + ACEI + BB + NIT + EVAL** **ADHF+ AFIB = SR + FUROS + ACEI + BB + REST-SR**
 DISCUSSION	Patients with diastolic heart failure have normal left ventricular ejection fraction and contractile function but have impaired relaxation and filling of the left ventricle.
 PEARLS	Mortality rate among patients with diastolic heart failure ranges from 5% to 8% annually (compared with 10–15% among patients with systolic heart failure).
 REFERENCE	1) Aurigemma GP, et al. Clinical practice. Diastolic heart failure. *N Engl J Med.* 2004;351:1097–1105. 2) Jessup M, et al. 2009 Focused update: ACCF/AHA guidelines for the diagnosis and management of heart failure in adults. *J Am Coll Cardiol.* 2009;53:1343–1382. 3) Angeja BG, et al. Evaluation and management of diastolic heart failure. *Circulation.* 2003;107:659. 4) Smith GL, Masoudi FA, Vaccarino V, Radford MJ, Krumholz HM. Outcomes in heart failure patients with preserved EF. *J Am Coll Cardiol.* 2003;41:1510–1581.

What is my congestive heart failure patient's New York Heart Association class?

KEY CONCEPT	Patient's congestive heart failure can be classified by presence of symptoms based upon the New York Heart Association classification.
HISTORY	HPI: Dyspnea on exertion or at rest, fatigue, weakness, diaphoresis. PMH: Hypertension, coronary artery disease, hyperlipidemia, diabetes, atrial fibrillation. PSH: Smoking, alcohol.
PHYSICAL EXAM	Peripheral edema, elevated jugular venous pressure, rales, laterally displaced apical impulse, S3 gallop.
IMAGING	ECHO: LVEF <40%, LA and LV enlargement, wall motion abnormalities. X-ray: Cardiomegaly, cephalization of pulmonary vessels (increased distribution of flow to apices), pleural effusion.
SYNTHESIS	**NYHA-I** = **N**ew **Y**ork **H**eart **A**ssociation class **I**. **NYHA-II** = **N**ew **Y**ork **H**eart **A**ssociation class **II**. **NYHA-III** = **N**ew **Y**ork **H**eart **A**ssociation class **III**. **NYHA-IV** = **N**ew **Y**ork **H**eart **A**ssociation class **IV**. **ASYMP** = **ASYMP**tomatic patient with ordinary physical activity not causing any fatigue, palpitations, dyspnea, or chest pain. **SYMP-STREN** = **SYMP**toms of fatigue, palpitations, dyspnea, or chest pain during **STREN**uous activity. **SYMP-ADL** = **SYMP**toms during **A**ctivities of **D**aily **L**iving. **SYMP-REST** = **SYMP**toms at **REST**, unable to carry out physical activity without discomfort.
EPIPHANY	**ASYMP = NYHA-I** **SYMP-STREN = NYHA-II** **SYMP-ADL = NYHA-III** **SYMP-REST = NYHA-IV**

DISCUSSION	The New York Heart Association classification system can be used to quantify congestive heart failure symptoms, facilitate communication between providers, prognosticate, and help in designing a treatment plan and making decisions regarding valve surgery, ICD placement, and medical therapy.
REFERENCE	1) Hunt SA, et al. 2009 focused update incorporated into the ACC/AHA 2005 guidelines for the diagnosis and management of heart failure in adults. *Circulation*. 2009;119:e391–e479.

How do I initially manage hypertensive emergency?

KEY CONCEPT	The management of hypertensive emergency is based on the associated clinical condition.
HISTORY	HPI: Symptoms of chest pain, headache, altered mental status, shortness of breath, cough, change in vision, back pain, oliguria. PMH: Hypertension, coronary artery disease, congestive heart failure, diabetes, chronic kidney disease. SH: Illicit drug use.
PHYSICAL EXAM	Blood pressure (BP) >180/120 mm Hg, new-onset murmur, retinal hemorrhage or exudates, rales, elevated JVP.
ELECTRO-CARDIOGRAM	ST elevation, ST depression, deep Q waves (>1 mm), poor R-wave progression.
SYNTHESIS	**HTNE** = **H**yper**T**e**N**sive **E**mergency: severe elevation in blood pressure (BP) >180/120 mm Hg. **HTNU** = **H**yper**T**e**N**sive **U**rgency: asymptomatic elevation in BP >160/100 mm Hg. **PULME** = **PULM**onary **E**dema. **AMIS** = **A**cute **M**yocardial **IS**chemia (angina, acute myocardial infarction). **AAD** = **A**cute **A**ortic **D**issection. **ARF** = **A**cute **R**enal **F**ailure. **ENC** = hypertensive **ENC**ephalopathy. **ECL** = **ECL**ampsia. **SC** = **S**ympathetic **C**risis: pheochromocytoma, autonomic dysfunction (post-spinal cord injury), drugs (cocaine, amphetamines, phenylpropanolamine, phencyclidine, or ingestion of MAOI and tyramine-containing food). **ESMO** = **ESMO**lol 80 mg bolus over 30 seconds followed by 150 mcg/kg/min IV. **HYD** = **HYD**ralazine IV bolus 5 mg, if BP does not decrease after 20 minutes repeat (maximum total dose 30 mg). **LOOP** = Furosemide 40 mg IV over 2 minutes. **NCD** = **N**i**C**ar**D**ipine 5 mg/hr IV. **LBTL** = **L**a**B**e**T**a**L**ol IV 2 mg/min (max 300 mg). **NTG** = **N**i**T**ro**G**lycerine 5 mcg/min IV. **NP** = **N**itro**P**russide 0.5 mcg/min IV.

E EPIPHANY	**HTNE + SC = NCD** **HTNE + ARF = NCD** **HTNE + PULME = NP + NG + LOOP** **HTNE + AAD = NP + ESMO** **HTNE + AMIS = NTG + LBTL** **HTNE + ENC = LBTL** **HTNE + ECL = HYD**
DISCUSSION	Hypertensive emergency is a serious condition that may result in end-organ damage if left untreated. Patients with HTNE should be transferred to an ICU setting and be treated immediately with IV antihypertensives with the goal of lowering the mean arterial pressure by 25% within the first hour.
CONTRA-INDICATIONS	– Nitroprusside is broken down into cyanide and can cause toxicity in patients on nitroprusside for prolonged periods of time. Monitor thiocyanate levels. – In patients with HTNE resulting from sympathetic crisis, beta blockers are contraindicated because inhibition of beta-receptor-induced vasodilation results in unopposed alpha-adrenergic vasoconstriction and a further rise in BP.
PEARLS	– A >20 mm Hg discrepancy in BP in both arms is suggestive of aortic dissection.
REFERENCE	1) Varon J, et al. The diagnosis and management of hypertensive crises. *Chest.* 2000;118:214–227.

How do I manage my patients elevated LDL level?

KEY CONCEPT	The management of a patient's low-density-lipoprotein level (LDL) is based on the presence of coronary artery disease (CAD), CAD equivalents, and risk factors.
HISTORY	HPI: Elevated LDL. PMH: CAD, diabetes mellitus, peripheral arterial disease, abdominal aortic aneurysm, hypertension, hyperlipidemia, transient ischemic attack (TIA), stroke. FH: Premature CAD (male first degree relatives <55 years, female first degree relative <65 years). SH: Smoking, alcohol.
PHYSICAL EXAM	Acanthosis nigricans, claudication, pale/cool extremities.
ELECTRO-CARDIOGRAM	ST depression, ST elevation, deep Q waves (>1 mm).

SYNTHESIS	**LDL** = Serum **L**ow-**D**ensity-**L**ipoprotein cholesterol level.
	CAD-EQ = Patient with **C**oronary **A**rtery **D**isease or CAD **EQ**uivalent: diabetes mellitus, peripheral artery disease, carotid artery disease (>50% stenosis), abdominal aortic aneurysm, multiple risk factors conferring a 10-year CAD risk of >20% (see Framingham risk score chapter). LDL goal is <70 mg/dL.
	2RF = Presence of >**2** of the following **R**isk **F**actors: hypertension, smoking, low high-density-lipoprotein (<40 mg/dL), family history of premature CAD, age (>=45 years male, >=55 years female); or a 10-year CAD risk of 1.0–20% (see Framingham risk score chapter). LDL goal is <130 mg/dL.
	01RF = Presence of **0** or **1** of the following **R**isk **F**actors: hypertension, smoking, low high-density-lipoprotein (<40 mg/dL), family history of premature CAD, age (>=45 years male, >=55 years female). LDL goal is <160 mg/dL.
	TLC = Recommend **T**herapeutic **L**ifestyle **C**hanges such as weight loss, aerobic exercise, and a diet low in fat, salt, and high in fiber.
	DT = Begin **D**rug **T**herapy with:
	  Atorvastatin 10 mg/day or
	  Lovastatin 40 mg/day or
	  Pravastatin 40 mg/day or
	  Simvastatin 20 mg/day
	  Fluvastatin 40 mg/day or
	  Rosuvastatin 5 mg/day or
	If unable to tolerate statins, then start gemfibrozil 600 mg BID and niacin 1.5 g/day.

EPIPHANY	**01RF + LDL>=160 = TLC** **01RF + LDL>=190 = DT** **2RF + LDL>=130 = TLC + DT** **CAD-EQ + LDL>=100 = TLC + DT**
DISCUSSION	Patients with CAD or a CAD equivalent require tight control with lifestyle modification and drug therapy with statins to prevent the progression of CAD.
CONTRA-INDICATIONS	– Statins can cause an elevation in aminotransaminases and should be discontinued in patients with in an increase >3 times the upper limit of normal. Patients with cholestasis or active liver disease should not be placed on statins. – Statins can produce a myopathy characterized by muscle aches, soreness, weakness, and elevated creatine kinase levels (>10 times the upper limit of normal), which can lead to rhabdomyolysis, myoglobinuria, and acute renal failure. If suspected or present, statin should be discontinued immediately.
PEARLS	– In patients with CAD and high cholesterol, statins have been shown to reduce the relative risk of major coronary events by 30%.
REFERENCE	1) Grundy SM, et al. Implications of recent clinical trials for the National Cholesterol Education Program Adult Treatment Panel III Guidelines. *Circulation*. 2004;110:227–39. 2) Pearson TA, et al. AHA guidelines for prevention of Cardiovascular disease. *Circulation*. 2002;106:388–391.

How do I manage my patients low HDL level?

KEY CONCEPT	The management of a patient's high-density-lipoprotein (HDL) levels is based on serum levels and presence of elevated low-density-lipoproteins (LDL).
HISTORY	HPI: Low HDL. PMH: Coronary artery disease (CAD), hypertension, hyperlipidemia, diabetes mellitus, metabolic syndrome. FH: Premature CAD (male first degree relatives <55 years, female first degree relative <65 years). SH: Smoking.
ELECTRO-CARDIOGRAM	ST depression, ST elevation, deep Q waves (>1 mm).
SYNTHESIS	**LOW-HDL** = **LOW** serum **HDL** < 40 mg/dL (men), HDL < 50 mg/dL (women); the optimal goal level to target is > = 60 mg/dL. **LS** = **L**ife**S**tyle changes: exercise, weight loss, smoking cessation. **NL-LDL** = **N**ormal **LDL** Level. **E-LDL** = **E**levated **LDL** (see chapter on managing LDL). **NCN** = Start either: **N**ia**C**i**N** extended release tablet at 500 mg once daily (given at bedtime) for 1 month; then increase dose by 500 mg each month to maximum of 2000 mg once daily. Or Niacin short acting 500 mg twice daily, titrating up to a maximum of 4500 mg/day. **INEFF-NCN** = **INEFF**ective **N**ia**C**i**N** or cannot tolerate niacin. **TL** = Treat elevated LDL (see chapter on managing LDL) first, then if HDL< 40 mg/dL give NCN and LS. **GEM** = **GEM**fibrozil 600 mg po BID.
E EPIPHANY	**LOW-HDL + NL-LDL = LS + NCN** **LOW-HDL + NL-LDL + INEFF-NCN = GEM** **LOW-HDL + E-LDL = TL**

DISCUSSION	Low levels of serum HDL increase the risk of CAD. Modification of lifestyle habits such as smoking and obesity which both decrease serum HDL can decrease the risk of morbidity and mortality from CAD. Patients should be advised to take niacin 30 minutes after taking their daily aspirin dose to reduce symptomatic side effects of niacin.
CONTRA-INDICATIONS	– Patients experiencing severe side effects of niacin (skin flushing, itching, dyspepsia) after 2 weeks should be placed on gemfibrozil 600 mg BID.
PEARLS	– Niacin (nicotinic acid) increases serum HDL levels by 15–35%. – Every 1% decrease in serum HDL is associated with a 2–3% increase in CAD.
REFERENCE	1) Third report of the National Cholesterol Education Program (NCEP) expert panel on detection, evaluation, and treatment of high blood cholesterol in adults. *Circulation.* 2002;106:3143.

How do I manage a patient with cardiogenic shock complicating a myocardial infarction?

KEY CONCEPT	The management of cardiogenic shock due to myocardial infarction is focused at stabilizing the patient for revascularization.
HISTORY	HPI: Recent symptoms of MI, altered mental status, sudden clinical decompensation. PMH: CAD, myocardial infarction, hypertension, hyperlipidemia, diabetes mellitus SH: Tobacco or cocaine use.
PHYSICAL EXAM	Hypotension (systolic BP < 80 mm Hg or mean arterial pressure 30 mm Hg below baseline), cool extremities, tachycardia, rales.
IMAGING	Pulmonary artery catheterization: Pulmonary capillary wedge pressure (PCWP) 15 mm Hg. ECHO: Ventricular function and wall motion, evidence of pericardial effusion, valve function. CXR: Cardiomegaly, pulmonary edema, pleural effusion.
SYNTHESIS (cont. on next page)	**CS-MI** = **C**ardiogenic **S**hock due to **M**yocardial **I**nfarction: To make diagnosis of cardiogenic shock must have hypotension [systolic BP < 80 mm Hg or mean arterial pressure 30 mm Hg below baseline]; cardiac index < 2.2 L/min/m^2; and PCWP > 15 mm Hg. For myocardial infarction, check for elevated cardiac biomarkers, electrocardiogram for ST changes or new Q-waves, and clinical history suggesting recent MI. **AC** = **A**nti**C**oagulate. For antiplatelet therapy, immediately give aspirin 325 mg chewed/swallowed. Start heparin infusion at 60 units/kg IV bolus followed by 12 units/kg/hr and titrate to keep PTT between 60–90 seconds. **STAB** = **STAB**ilize. Give 1 liter fluid bolus if hypotensive. If inadequate response, start dopamine infusion at 5 mcg/kg/min and titrate to MAP > 60 mm Hg. If dopamine causes severe tachycardia, use norepinephrine instead. If unable to achieve adequate blood pressure with inotropes, place intra-aortic ballon pump emergently. Place an arterial line to titrate inotropes. Patients will usually require mechanical ventilation. **RVS** = **ReVaS**cularization: Coronary angiography and then mechanical revascularization with PCI or CABG is optimal. The earlier revascularization is performed, the better the outcome. **FLUID** = Fix **FLUID** status. In patients with persistent hypotension after an empiric fluid bolus, place a pulmonary artery (Swan-Ganz) catheter to guide inotrope use and fluid management. Keep the pulmonary capillary wedge pressure < 20 mm Hg. Patients will often need dieresis despite being hypotensive.

SYNTHESIS (cont. from previous page)	**MED-TX** = Medical management. Admit to intensive care. Revascularization gives the greatest chance of recovering myocardial function. Reduce afterload (such as with ACE-Inhibitors) and attempt to wean off inotropes and balloon pump support. As fluid status corrected and pulmonary edema improves, attempt to wean from mechanical ventilation. If left with severe cardiac dysfunction, patient will need evaluation by a heart failure/transplant specialist and may be candidate for advanced heart failure treatments such as a ventricular assist device.
EPIPHANY	**CS-MI = STAB + AC + RVS + FLUID + MED-TX**
DISCUSSION	The most common cause of cardiogenic shock is acute myocardial infarction with left ventricular dysfunction. Other less common causes of cardiogenic shock such as aortic dissection, papillary muscle rupture, ventricular septal rupture, or cardiac tamponade are managed differently and not detailed in this chapter.
CONTRA-INDICATIONS	– An intra-aortic balloon pump should not be placed in patients with severe aortic regurgitation.
PEARLS	– Cardiogenic shock occurs in 5–8% of patients hospitalized with STEMI and 2.5% of NSTEMI cases. – Left ventricular ejection fraction < 28% is associated with a higher mortality in patients with cardiogenic shock.
REFERENCE	1) Reynolds HR, et al. Cardiogenic shock: current concepts and improving outcomes. *Circulation*. 2008;117:686–697. 2) Picard MH, et al. Echocardiographic predictors of survival and response to early revascularization in cardiogenic shock *Circulation*. 2003;107(2): 279–284.

Does my patient have metabolic syndrome?

KEY CONCEPT	The diagnosis of metabolic syndrome is based upon the presence of a cluster of certain risk factors, physical findings, and laboratory results.
HISTORY	HPI: Obese individual with elevated blood glucose and lipids. PMH: Coronary artery disease (CAD), diabetes, hyperlipidemia, hypertension, obesity. FH: Premature CAD (male first degree relatives <55 years, female first degree relative <65 years), obesity. SH: Smoking, alcohol.
PHYSICAL EXAM	Central obesity, acanthosis nigricans (hyperpigmentation of skin found in body folds of skin), claudication, pale/cool extremities.
SYNTHESIS	**MET-SD** = **MET**abolic **S**yn**D**rome. **ELEV-BP** = **ELEV**ated **B**lood **P**ressure >130/85 mm Hg or on drug treatment for hypertension. **ELEV-FG** = **ELEV**ated **F**asting **G**lucose > 100 mg/dL. **C-OBES** = Abdominal **C**entral **OBES**ity: waist for men >40 inches (102 cm) and women >35 inches (88 cm). **TRIG** = Elevated **TRIG**lycerides >150 mg/dL. **LOW-HDL** = **LOW HDL**: men <40 mg/dL, women <50 mg/dL. **3-FAC** = Patient with more than three of the following **FAC**tors: ELEV-BP, ELEV-FG, C-OBES, TRIG, or LOW-HDL.
EPIPHANY	**3-FAC = MET-SD**
DISCUSSION	Metabolic syndrome is a constellation of disorders that can promote the development of atherosclerotic cardiovascular disease. Patients who are at risk should be evaluated in the clinic setting, and the appropriate lifestyle modifications should be instituted.

PEARLS	– The predominant risk factors behind metabolic syndrome are abdominal obesity and insulin resistance.
REFERENCE	1) Grundy SM, et al. Diagnosis and management of metabolic syndrome. *Circulation.* 2005;112:2735–2752 2) Expert Panel on Detection, Evaluation, and Treatment of High Blood Cholesterol in Adults. Executive summary of the third report of The National Cholesterol Education Program (NCEP) expert panel on detection, evaluation, and treatment of high blood cholesterol in adults (Adult Treatment Panel III). *JAMA.* 2001;285:2486.

How do I manage my patient with metabolic syndrome?

KEY CONCEPT	The management of metabolic syndrome is based upon lifestyle modification and pharmacological control of risk factors.
HISTORY	HPI: Obese individual with elevated blood glucose and lipids. PMH: Coronary artery disease (CAD), diabetes, hyperlipidemia, hypertension, obesity. FH: Premature CAD [male first degree relatives < 55 years, female first degree relative < 65 years], obesity. SH: Smoking, alcohol.
PHYSICAL EXAM	Central obesity, acanthosis nigricans (hyperpigmentation of skin found in body folds of skin), claudication, pale/cool extremities.
SYNTHESIS	**MET-SD** = Patient diagnosed with **MET**abolic **S**yn**D**rome (see the chapter "Does my patient have metabolic syndrome?"). **WL10** = **W**eight **L**oss 7–**10**% in first year, continued weight loss afterwards with goal of body mass index (BMI) of < 25 kg/m². **EXER** = At least 30 minutes of continuous or intermittent moderate intensity **EXER**cise 5 times per week. **DIET** = **DIET** should have saturated fat < 7% of total calories, dietary cholesterol < 200 mg/day, total fat is 25–35% of total calories. **ELEV-GLUC** = For patient with impaired fasting glucose (fasting glucose 100–125 mg/dL) encourage physical activity and weight reduction (7–10% weight loss in first year with continued weight loss afterward with target BMI of < 25 kg/m²); for patients with type 2 diabetes institute lifestyle modifications and pharmacotherapy with goal of HbA1C < 7%. **DYS-LIP** = For patients with **DYSLIP**idemia, see chapter on LDL and HDL treatment. **ELEV-BP** = For **ELEV**ated **B**lood **P**ressure, reduce blood pressure with goal of 140/90 mm Hg (130/80 mm Hg in diabetics). Give lisinopril 10 mg/day; if cannot folerate ACE inhibitor, give losartan 25 mg/day. **ASP** = Low dose **ASP**irin 81 mg/day.
E EPIPHANY	**MET-SD = WL10 + EXER + DIET + ELEV GLUC + DYS-LIP + ELEV BP + ASP**

 DISCUSSION	The primary goal in management of metabolic syndrome is to decrease the risk of clinical atherosclerotic cardiovascular disease.
 PEARLS	– Glycemic control to a hemoglobin A1C of <7% reduces microvascular complications and may decrease the risk for macrovascular disease as well.
 REFERENCE	1) Grundy SM, et al. Diagnosis and management of metabolic syndrome. *Circulation.* 2005;112:2735–2752. 2) Expert Panel on Detection, Evaluation, and Treatment of High Blood Cholesterol in Adults. Executive summary of the third report of The National Cholesterol Education Program (NCEP) expert panel on detection, evaluation, and treatment of high blood cholesterol in adults (Adult Treatment Panel III). *JAMA.* 2001;285:2486.

How do I manage a patient with labile blood pressure?

KEY CONCEPT	Subcategory of hypertension with abrupt fluctuations in blood pressure levels and sympathetic activation.
HISTORY	Patients present with headache, chest pain, dizziness, nausea and vomiting, palpitations, flushing, and diaphoresis and can be during anxious/stressful situation.
	Anxiety disorders, salt sensitivity, stress, caffeine, drugs, medical disorders (pheochromocytoma, carcinoid syndrome).
PHYSICAL EXAM	Ranges from normal to end stage manifestations of hypertension.
ELECTRO-CARDIOGRAM	ECG: Can be normal or tachycardia during states of stress.
IMAGING	CT/MRI head to rule out stroke, tumor, hemorrhage, brainstem compression, trauma.
	CT abdomen to rule out adrenal masses.
	Carotid ultrasound to rule out stenosis that can cause barorecepter failure.
	Renal ultrasound to rule out stenosis.
SYNTHESIS (cont. on next page)	**LAB-HTN** = patient with **LAB**ile **H**yper**T**e**N**sion
	ANX = **ANX**iety/stress.
	SS = **S**alt **S**ensitivity.
	DRUG = Caffeine/**DRUG**s.
	PHEO = **PHEO**chromocytoma.
	CS = **C**arcinoid **S**yndrome.
	HT = **H**yper**T**hyroidism.
	RHTN = **R**enovascular **H**yper**T**e**N**sion, renal artery stenosis.
	BR = **B**aroreceptor **R**eflex/autonomic dysfunction.
	LC = **L**ifestyles **C**hanges (salt and fat reduction/weight loss).
	SR = **S**tress **R**eduction (benzodiazepines/antidepressants/stress management/biofeedback).
	DM = **D**rug **M**odification (reduce consumption/diet modification/withdraw offending drug).
	HM = **H**ypertensive **M**edication (alpha/beta blockade metoprolol and prazosin, clonidine).
	OS = **O**ctreotide and **S**urgery.
	ACEI = **ACE**-Inhibitors, stents, surgery.

SYNTHESIS (cont. from previous page)	**ATM** = AntiThyroid Medication (PTU or methimazole, surgery if indicated). **SFME** = Supportive Fludrocortisones, Midodrine, Ephedrine, SSRI. **S** = Surgery. **ADR** = ADRenal mass.
E EPIPHANY	**LAB-HTN + ANX = SR** **LAB-HTN + SS = LC** **LAB-HTN + DRUG = DM** **LAB-HTN + PHEO = HM** **LAB-HTN + CS = OS** **LAB-HTN + HT = ATM** **LAB-HTN + RHTN = ACEI** **LAB-HTN + BR = SFME** **LAB-HTN + ADR = S**
DISCUSSION	Episodes of paroxysmal hypertension can last minutes to hours and between the pressures can be normal.
PEARLS	– Pseudopheochromocytoma is characterized by autonomic manifestations (ie, paroxysmal hypertension). – Panic disorder is characterized by emotional manifestations, and blood pressure changes are milder.
REFERENCE	1) Mann DF. Severe paroxysmal hypertension. *Arch Intern Med.* 1999159:670. 2) Mackenzie IS, Brown MJ. Pseudopheochromocytoma. *J Hypertens.* 2007;25:2204. 3) Juchel O, Buu NT, Hamet P, et al. Dopamine surges in hyperadrenergic essential hypertension. *Hypertension.* 1982;4:845.

How should I initially work up my patient with syncope?

 KEY CONCEPT	A transient loss of consciousness due to temporary cerebral hypoperfusion.
 HISTORY	HPI: Brief loss of consciousness, palpitations, blurred vision, nausea, diaphoresis, light headedness, fatigue. PMHx/PSxHx: Number of attacks, seizures, TIA, pacemaker/defi brillators. Social/Fhx: heart disease, stroke, alcohol/substance abuse/cocaine/sedatives, fear or emotional culprits, positional. Meds: Diuretics, antihypertensives, beta-blockers, antidepressants.
 PHYSICAL EXAM	PE: Vitals and orthostatic pulse and blood pressure. Complete cardiac exam. Complete neuro exam.
 IMAGING	ECG: Heart block, arrhythmias. Echo/valve defects, ejection fraction for CHF, CXR for pneumonia, edema, PE.
SYNTHESIS (cont. on next page)	**SY** = Patient presenting with **SY**ncope. **ANEMIA** = Check for **ANEMIA** & transfuse/work up as clinically indicated. **LOW-BSL** = Check for **LOW B**lood **S**ugar (glucose) **L**evel & work up. **STOP-MED** = If patient is bradycardic, **STOP** all **MED**ications that affect cardiac conduction, eg, beta blockers, calcium-channel blockers. **ORTHO** = Check for **ORTHO**statics. ie, check for drop in BP of >=20 mm Hg systolic or 10 mm Hg diastolic within 3 minutes of standing. **ORTHO-POS/ORTHO-NEG** = **POS**itive for/**NEG**ative for **ORTHO**statics. **ECG** = Perform 12-lead **ECG**. **ECG-POS** = **ECG** is **POS**itive for conduction conditions associated with syncope eg, Sinus node dysfunction (sinus arrest > 3 seconds); second or third-degree heart block; supraventricular tachycardia, ventricular tachycardia; pacemaker/implantable cardioverter-defibrillator malfunction, torsade de point. **ECG-NEG** = **ECG** is **NEG**ative for conditions associated with syncope. **LSM** = **L**oud **S**ystolic **M**urmur on physical exam. **LSM-NEG** = **L**oud **S**ystolic **M**urmur **NEG**ative on physical exam. **SY-TURN** = **SY**ncope with head **TURN**, shaving, or wearing a tight collar. **CSM** = Patient upright, begin with the right carotid artery; use firm longitudinal massage with increasing pressure for 5 seconds. **CSM-POS** = **C**arotid **S**inus **M**assage **POS**itive: produces paroxysmal atrioventricular block or asystole of >=3 seconds duration, or fall in BP from baseline of 50 mm Hg systolic or 30 mm Hg diastolic, and occurrence of syncope or presyncope symptoms. **CSM-NEG** = **C**arotid **S**inus **M**assage **NEG**ative.

SYNTHESIS (cont. from previous page)

SY-ORTHO = ORTHOstatic **SY**ncope = Evaluate and treat the underlying cause [volume depletion (tachycardia and a heart rate >100 beats per minute), barorefl ex impairment (minimal cardiac acceleration in older patients), medications (antihypertensives, antidepressants, diuretics), and autonomic insufficiency (diabetes mellitus, amyloid neuropathy, Parkinson's disease, multiple system atrophy, alcohol abuse).

CBV-SYS = Patient manifesting signs/symptoms of **C**ere**B**ro**V**ascular diseases at time of **SYN**copal episode, eg, transient ischemic attack, seizure, migraine, subclavian steal syndrome.

NCGS = **N**euro**C**ardio**G**enic **S**yncope.

CARS = **CAR**diac **S**yncope.

RFMS = **R**e**F**lex **M**ediated **S**yncope eg, Vasovagal syncope (common faint), carotid sinus hypersensitivity, situational (coughing, sneezing, defecating, micturition, postmicturition), or glossopharyngeal and trigeminal neuralgia.

CBVS = **C**ere**B**ro**V**ascular **S**yncope: recommend consult neurology for further work up as clinically indicated.

PA-DI = Symptoms of **PAL**pitations and **DI**zziness.

HOLT = Get 24-hour **HOLT**er monitor.

HOLT-POS = **HOLT**er monitor (or telemetry) is **POS**itive for sinus node dysfunction (sinus arrest >3 seconds); second- or third-degree heart block; supraventricular tachycardia, ventricular tachycardia; pacemaker/implantable cardioverter-defi brillator malfunction, torsade de point.

HOLT-NEG = **HOLT**er monitor (or telemetry) is **NEG**ative for arrhythmia.

EVENT = evaluation with **EVENT** recorder or implantable loop recorder.

ECHO = Get **ECHO**cardiogram.

ECHO-POS = **ECHO**cardiogram **POS**itive for significant structural heart disease associated with syncope, eg, aortic stenosis, mitral stenosis, acute coronary syndromes/ischemia, pulmonary embolism, pulmonary hypertension, acute aortic dissection, hypertrophic cardiomyopathy, pericardial effusion/tamponade, atrial myxoma.

ECHO-NEG = **ECHO**cardiogram **NEG**ative for significant heart disease.

CST = get **C**ardiac **S**tress **T**est.

CST-POS/CST-NEG = **C**ardiac **S**tress **T**est **POS**itive/**NEG**ative significant ischemia.

TUC = **T**reat **U**nderlying **C**ause and/or referral for electrophysiology study, catheterization, or surgery if clinically indicated.

 EPIPHANY	SY = STOP-MED + ANEMIA + LOW-BSL + ORTHO + ECG + HOLT + ECHO + CSM + CST SY-TURN = CSM SY-TURN + CSM-POS = TUC SY + HOLT-NEG + ORTHO-NEG + CSM-NEG + ECHO-NEG + CST-NEG = RFMS SY + ORTHO = SY-ORTHO SY + CBV-SYS = CBVS SY + LSM = ECHO + HOLT SY + ECHO-POS = CARS SY + HOLT-POS = CARS SY + CST-POS = CARS CARS = TUC
 REFERENCE	1) Brignole M, et al. Guidelines on management (diagnosis and treatment) of syncope. *Eur Heart J.* 2001;22:1290. 2) Miller TH, et al. Evaluation of syncope. *Am Fam Physician.* 2005;72:1492–1500.

MEDICATIONS

When should I evaluate cardiac function in my patient about to receive or currently receiving doxorubicin?

KEY CONCEPT	In patients receiving doxorubicin chemotherapy, monitoring of cardiac function is based upon baseline left ventricular function and total chemotherapy dosage received.
IMAGING	HPI: Patient with Hodgkin's lymphoma, breast, bladder, stomach, or lung cancer receiving chemotherapy with doxorubicin. PMH: Congestive heart failure, hypertension, coronary artery disease. SH: Alcohol.
PHYSICAL EXAM	Dyspnea, rales, tachycardia, jugular–venous distention, hepatomegaly, edema of ankle. Acute toxicity: Arrhythmias, electrocardiographic abnormalities, a pericarditis–myocarditis syndrome, and ventricular dysfunction during or immediately after administration of anthracyclines. Early toxicity: Observed as dose-related occurrence of CHF in pts that received 500–550 mg/m^2 of doxorubicin. Late toxicity: The onset of symptomatic CHF can occur as late as 10–12 years after the last anthracycline dose. Late CHF is due to a nonischemic dilated cardiomyopathy.
IMAGING	ECHO: LVEF <40%, LA and LV enlargement, wall motion abnormalities. Radionuclide angiography (RNA): Monitoring changes in diastolic left ventricular function may identify evidence of cardiotoxicity earlier than monitoring ejection fraction, which is a marker of systolic function.
SYNTHESIS	**B4DOX** = **B**efore patient receives **DOX**orubicin or prior to administration of 100 mg/m^2 of doxorubicin. **PTDOX** = **Pa**Tient has already received >100 mg/m^2 **DOX**orubicin. **EF-EVAL** = Refer patient for echocardiogram, radionuclide angiography, or other imaging test for left ventricular **E**jection **F**raction **EVAL**uation. **LVEF-OK** = **LVEF** normal or if follow-up study shows decline in less that 10% from baseline study and absolute EF >= 30%. **LVEF<30** = **LVEF <30**%. **DECL-10** = LVEF **DECL**ines by **10**% from baseline study. **DC-DOX** = **D**is**C**ontinue **DOX**orubicin. **CON-DOX** = **CON**tinue **DOX**orubicin. **FU-#1** = **F**ollow-**U**p study **#1** with EF-EVAL at 300 mg/m^2. Repeat EF-EVAL at 400 mg/m^2 if patient has history of cardiomyopathy, radiation exposure, and abnormal electrocardiographic results, or is on cyclophosphamide therapy. **FU-#2** = **F**ollow-**U**p study **#2** with EF-EVAL at 450 mg/m^2. **FU-#3** = **F**ollow-**U**p study **#3** with EF-EVAL prior to each dose after 450 mg/m^2.

E EPIPHANY	**B4DOX = EF-EVAL** **FU-#1 = EF-EVAL** **FU-#2 = EF-EVAL** **FU-#3 = EF-EVAL** **PTDOX + LVEF-OK = CON-DOX** **PTDOX + LVEF<30 = DC-DOX** **PTDOX + DECL-10 = DC-DOX**
DISCUSSION	The mechanism of doxorubicin cardiomyopathy may be due to the generation of free radicals and oxidative stress causing subcellular changes in the myocardium leading to loss of myofibrils and vacuolization of myocardial cells.
PEARLS	– Endomyocardial biopsy has the highest sensitivity and specificity for the diagnosis of doxorubicin-induced cardiomyopathy. – Patients with age >65 are predisposed to cardiotoxicity at lower cumulative doses of doxorubicin.
REFERENCE	1) Singal PK. Doxorubicin-induced cardiomyopathy. *N Engl J Med.* 1998; 339:900–905. 2) Schwartz RG, et al. Congestive heart failure and left ventricular dysfunction complicating doxorubicin therapy. *Am J Med.*1987;82(6):1109–1118. 3) Lee BH, Goodenday LS, Muswick GJ, et al. Alterations in left ventricular diastolic function with doxorubicin therapy. *J Am Coll Cardiol.* 1987;9:184.

What is the difference between all the beta blockers?

KEY CONCEPT	Beta blockers are used for many different conditions. The profiles of each beta blocker are important to make the best management decision for your patient.
HISTORY	A patient who presents with angina and a beta blocker is chosen for therapy.
PHYSICAL EXAM	Make note of signs of liver and kidney disease to monitor doses based on route of elimination; if positive asthma/COPD use of cardioselective agents, diabetes (can facilitate hypoglycemia and mask its effects).
ELECTRO-CARDIOGRAM	Monitor for 1st degree AV block, bradycardia.
SYNTHESIS	**ACE** = Acebutol **ATE** = ATEnolol **BET** = BETaxolol **BIOP** = BIOProlol. **CART** = CARTeolol **CARV** = CARVedilol **ESM** = ESMolol **LABE** = LABEtaolol **MET** = METoprolol **NAD** = NADolol. **NEB** = NEBivolol **OX** = OXprenolol **PEN** = PENbutolol. **PIND** = PINDolol **PROP** = PROPranolol **SOT** = SOTalol **TIM** = TIMolol. **AB** = **A**lpha **B**lock. **NAB** = **N**o **A**lpha **B**lock. **BS** = **B**eta **S**elective. **NBS** = **N**on-**B**eta **S**elective. **RE** = **R**enal **E**limination. **HE** = **H**epatic **E**limination.
E EPIPHANY (cont. on next page)	**ACE:** NAB, mild BS, dose 100–400 mg BID, half life 3–4 hours, HE **ATE:** NAB, high BS, dose 50–200 mg daily, half life 6–9 hours, RE **BET:** NAD, mild BS, dose, 10–20 mg daily, half life 9–12 hours, HE **BIOP:** NAB, mild BS, dose 2.5–20 mg daily, half life 9–12 hours, RE **CART:** NAB, NBS, dose 2.5–5 mg daily, half life 6 hours, RE **CARV:** AB, NBS, dose 2.125–25 mg BID, half life 7–10 hours, HE **ESM:** NAD, high BS, IV dose 500 mcg/kg/min titrate, half life 9 minutes, blood esterase elimination **LABE:** AB, NBS, dose 100–400 mg BID, half life 3–4 hours, HE **MET:** NAB, BS, dose 25–100 mg BID/TID, half life 3–7 hours, HE **NAD:** NAB, NBS, dose 40–160 mg daily, half life 24 hours, RE **NEB:** NAB, BS, dose 5–40 mg daily, half life 12 hours, HE **OX:** NAB, NBS, dose 40–80 mg TID, half life 1.5 hours, HE

E EPIPHANY (cont. from previous page)	**PEN: NAB, NBS, dose 10–40 mg daily, half life 5 hours, HE** **PIND: NAB, NBS, dose 5–30 mg, half life 3–4 hours, HE** **PROP: NAB, NBS, dose 10–80 mg BID/TID/QID, half life 3–4 hours, HE** **SOT: NAB, NBS, 80–160 mg BID, half life 12 hours, RE, independent class III antiarrhythmic activity** **TIM: NAB, NBS, dose10–30 mg BID, half life 4 hours, HE**
DISCUSSION	Beta blockers have shown to improve survival in patients with prior myocardial infarction and systolic heart failure. Beta blockers are used for angina, atrial fibrillation, heart failure, essential tremors, glaucoma, hypertension, migraines, aortic dissection, anxiety, portal hypertension, and various other uses.
PEARLS	– Sotalol also has antiarrhythmic activity. – Carvedilol and labetalol are only ones that have alpha blockade. – Propranolol and metoprolol enter the CNS in high concentrations and can have CNS side effects. – They are all equally effective in treating angina. – Oxprenolol, pindolol, acebutolol, and penbutolol are partial agonists and have simpathomimetic activity (good for patients with bradycardia, but not for post-myocardial infarction patients).
REFERENCE	1) Freemantle N, et al. Beta Blockade after myocardial infarction: systematic review and meta regression analysis. *BMJ.* 1999;318(7200):1730–1737. 2) Frishman WH, et al. *Current Cardiovascular Drugs.* Philadelphia: Current Medicine LLC; 2005.

Management of anticoagulation in patients on warfarin going for surgery?

 KEY CONCEPT	Interruption of anticoagulation increases the thromboembolic (TE) risk, while continuing it increases the surgical bleeding (SB) risk.
 HISTORY	HPI: Patient on warfarin undergoing surgery
 PHYSICAL EXAM	High TE Risk: Mechanical click.
 SURGERY	**HIGH-SBR = HIGH SB R**isk: neurosurgery, genitourinary, cardiothoracic, major vascular (AAA repair, aortofemoral bypass), major urologic (prostatectomy, bladder tumor resection), major orthopedic (hip/knee replacement), lung resection surgery, intestinal anastomosis surgery, permanent pacemaker or ICD insertion, miscellaneous (kidney–prostate–cervical cone biopsy, pericardiocentesis, colonic polypectomy). **INT-SBR = INT**ermediate **SB R**isk: other intraabdominal, intrathoracic, orthopedic, or vascular surgery. **LOW-SBR = LOW SB R**isk: laparoscopic cholecystectomy/inguinal herniorrhaphy, dental procedures, skin excisions, endoscopy/colonoscopy, ophthalmologic procedures, coronary angiography, bone marrow aspiration/biopsy, lymph node biopsy, thoracocentesis, paracentesis, arthrocentesis.
 SYNTHESIS	**HIGH-TER = HIGH-TE R**isk: mechanical heart valve, arterial thromboembolism within 3 months (stroke, transient ischemic attack [TIA], systemic embolism), venous thromboembolism within 3 months (DVT, PE), prior arterial/venous thromboembolism during interruption of warfarin, prothrombotic condition (protein C, S, or antithrombin deficiency, antiphospholipid antibodies, multiple prothrombotic blood abnormalities). **INT-TER = INT**ermediate **TE R**isk: bioprosthetic heart valve, chronic atrial fibrillation with at least 1 major stroke risk factor (congestive heart failure, hypertension, age >75, diabetes, prior stroke/TIA), prior arterial/venous thromboembolism within past 3–12 months. **LOW-TER = LOW TE R**isk: chronic atrial fibrillation with no major risk factors, prior arterial/venous thromboembolism over 12 months ago.

 E EPIPHANY	**HIGH-TER/INT-TER + HIGH-SBR/INT-SBR = Stop warfarin 5 days prior to surgery, with surgery day target International Normalized Ratio (INR) <=1.5 (<=2.0 with mechanical valves). Begin intravenous unfractionated heparin (IV-UFH) with bolus or low-molecular-weight heparin (LMWH) 3 days prior to surgery. If the INR on day of surgery is >1.5 (>=2.0 with mechanical valves), give 1 mg subcutaneous vitamin K. Stop IV-UFH 5 hours (LMWH 24 hours) prior to surgery. Restart heparin with no bolus/ LMWH 12 hours after surgery and warfarin day 1 post surgery (wait longer if bleeding from surgical site or not taking PO). HIGH-TER/INT-TER + LOW-SBR = No interruption of warfarin. LOW-TER + HIGH-SBR/ INT-SBR = Stop warfarin 5 days prior to surgery with surgery day target INR <=1.5 (<=2.0 with mechanical valves). Bridge with pre- and post-operative UFH prophylaxis 5000 U subcutaneously q12h (or LMWH). If INR on day of surgery is >1.5 (>=2.0 with mechanical valves) give 1 mg SC vitamin K. Restart prophylaxis 12 hours after surgery and warfarin day 1 post-surgery (wait longer if bleeding from surgical site or not taking PO).**
 DISCUSSION	Risk of recurrent events off therapy: Up to 18% with atrial fibrillation, up to 40% with thromboembolic events, up to 91% with mechanical valves (mitral > aortic).
 PEARLS	– Check INR day of surgery (or 24 hours preoperatively). – Graduated compression stockings or intermittent pneumatic compression can be added to reduce TE risk.
 REFERENCE	1) Bonow RO, et al. ACC/AHA 2008 guideline update on valvular heart disease: focused update on infective endocarditis. *J Am Coll Cardiol.* 2006;48:e1.

What are the surgical perioperative management indications with aspirin?

KEY CONCEPT	Aspirin use must be balanced between decreasing cardiovascular risk and increasing perioperative bleeding risk.
HISTORY	**HPI:** When and what type of surgery is planned. **PMH:** CAD, MI, vascular stents that have been placed (when and what type), thromboembolic events (ex. stroke), prosthetic valves. **SH:** Tobacco use.
SYNTHESIS	**LCER = Low Cardiovascular Event Risk:** Aspirin is taken prophylactically prior to prevent a first cardiovascular event. **HCER = High Cardiovascular Event Risk:** Aspirin is taken as secondary prevention in a patient with established cardiovascular disease (history of obstructive coronary artery disease, myocardial infarction, stroke, peripheral vascular disease). **UCER = Ultra High Cardiovascular Event Risk:** Includes: Patient had a recent stent placed (bare metal stent within the last 6 weeks or drug eluting stent within last 12 months). Patient with stent in the left main or left anterior descending coronary artery. Patient with a history of in-stent thrombosis. **LSB = Low Surgical Bleeding Risk:** Hemorrhage would likely not affect outcome. Examples: Dental procedures, skin excisions, endoscopy, ophthalmologic procedures, arthrocentesis, percutaneous coronary intervention. **HSB = High Surgical Bleeding Risk:** Hemorrhage could be catastrophic. Examples: Neurosurgery, orthopedic, genitourinary. **STOP = STOP** aspirin: Stop aspirin 7–10 days prior to surgery and resume 24 hours postoperatively when adequate hemostasis has occurred. **TAKE** = Continue to **TAKE** aspirin through procedure. **EVAL** = Careful **EVAL**uation of risks versus benefits. These patients are at extreme risk for a catastrophic event such as an acute thrombosis of a stent that can be fatal or cause permanent severe heart failure. Discussion should be made with patient, anesthesiologist, and surgeon. Timing of the surgery may have to be delayed if recent stent. If aspirin is stopped it should be clear that risk is extremely high.
E **EPIPHANY**	**LCER + LSB = TAKE** **LCER + HSB = STOP** **HCER + LSB = TAKE** **HCER + HSB = STOP** **UCER + LSB = TAKE** **UCER + HSB = EVAL**

DISCUSSION	Many patients in the UCER category are unaware of how catastrophic stopping anti-platelet medicine can be. Various medical specialties may give generic instructions to stop aspirin to all patients before medical procedures. UCER patients should have clear instructions to discuss with their cardiologist if ever instructed to stop aspirin for an elective procedure.
PEARLS	– Direct communication with the patient, anesthesiologist, and surgeon is very helpful to understand the surgical risk and make an informed decision.
REFERENCE	1) Douketis, et al. The perioperative management of antithrombotic therapy. *Chest.* 2008;133:299S–339S. 2) Bhattt DL, et al. ACCF/ACG/AHA 2008 expert consensus document of reducing the gastrointestinal risks of antiplatelet therapy and NSAID use. *Circulation.* 2008;118:1894.

How do I manage an elevated INR in a patient on warfarin?

KEY CONCEPT	INR is a ratio of the patient's prothrombin time to a normal control sample. A high value indicates higher chance of bleeding and a low value indicates higher chance of clotting.
HISTORY	HPI: Patient with elevated INR, bleeding and/or need for urgent reversal (prior to procedure). PMH: Atrial fibrillation, bioprosthetic heart valve, deep venous thrombosis, pulmonary embolism, prothrombotic condition [protein C, S or antithrombin deficiency]. SH: Alcohol intake, dietary vitamin K.
PHYSICAL EXAM	Bruising, bleeding, melena, dental bleeding, hematuria.
SYNTHESIS	**ST-INR = S**upratherapeutic **INR**: > 3.0; > 3.5 [mechanical heart valve] **SB = S**erious **B**leed – melena, hemoptysis, intravenous catheter bleeding, significant drop in hemoglobin, intracranial bleed. **NSB = N**o **S**erious **B**leeding
EPIPHANY	**SB = Hold warfarin and give vitamin K 10 mg by slow IV infusion. If bleeding continues, transfuse fresh frozen plasma (FFP).** **ST-INR ≥ 9 + NSB = Hold warfarin and give oral vitamin K 5.0 mg. Restart warfarin at a lower dose when INR is in therapeutic range.** **ST-INR 5 to <9 + NSB = Hold 1 or 2 doses of warfarin, then restart at lower dose. Give 2.5 mg of oral vitamin K in patients with high risk of bleeding. Restart warfarin at a lower dose when INR is in therapeutic range.** **ST-INR < 5 + NSB = Lower warfarin dose or hold 1 dose. Restart warfarin at a lower dose when INR is in therapeutic range.**
DISCUSSION	Therapeutic INR: 2–3; 2.5–3.5 (mechanical heart valve). In patients with supratherapeutic INR levels, warfarin doses must be lowered to allow INR to fall back to therapeutic levels to prevent the risk of serious bleeding. Patients with subtherapeutic INR run the risk of poor anticoagulation and thrombosis.
CONTRA-INDICATIONS	– Drug interactions that increase INR: acetaminophen, amiodarone, cimetidine, erythromycin, ketoconazole, metronidazole, propafenone, trimethoprim-sulfomethoxazole. – Drug interactions that decrease INR: barbiturates, rifampin, azathioprine, carbamazepine, cholestyramine.

PEARLS

– Blood samples taken from a central venous catheter can result in falsely elevated INRs due to heparin contamination; draw blood from a peripheral vein.

REFERENCE

1) Ansall J, Hirsh J, Hylek E. Guidelines for correction of warfarin over-anticoagulation. *Chest.* 2008;133:160–198.
2) Hylek EM, Heiman H, Skates SJ, Sheehan MA, Singer DE, et al. Acetominophen and other risk factors for excessive warfarin anticoagulation. *JAMA.* 1998;279:657–662.

How much protamine sulfate do I need to give to reverse heparin anticoagulation?

KEY CONCEPT	Reversal of heparin anticoagulation is done with protamine sulfate based on the time elapsed from the last dose of heparin.
HISTORY	HPI = Patient on low-molecular-weight or unfractionated heparin who is in need of reversal (prior to procedure, life-threatening bleed). PMH: Deep venous thrombosis (DVT), pulmonary embolus, unstable angina, non-ST-elevation myocardial infarction (NSTEMI).
SYNTHESIS	**HEP-PT** = **HEP**arinized **Pa**Tient who needs reversal of their anticoagulation. **PS** = **P**rotamine **S**ulfate is used to reverse heparin anticoagulation by binding to heparin in the blood and forming a stable complex. Should be administered by slow IV dose at a rate not >5 mg/min with a maximum dose of 50 mg. **T1** = Immediately after administration of heparin. **T2** = 30–60 minutes after administration of heparin. **T3** = >2 hours after administration of heparin. **P1** = 1 mg IV of PS per 100 units of heparin. **P2** = 0.5 mg IV of PS per 100 units of heparin. **P3** = 0.25 mg IV of per 100 units of heparin.
EPIPHANY	**HEP-PT + T1 = P1** **HEP-PT + T2 = P2** **HEP-PT + T3 = P3**
DISCUSSION	The recommended dose of protamine sulfate is 1 mg per 100 units of heparin, but this dose is adjusted based on the time since the last dose of heparin. The half life of heparin is 1.5 hours.
CONTRA-INDICATIONS	– Rapid infusion of protamine sulfate (>5 mg/min) can result in hypotension, anaphylactoid reaction (dyspnea, bradycardia, flushing), pulmonary hypertension, lassitude, nausea, and vomiting.

PEARLS

– Protamine sulfate neutralizes 60% of the anticoagulant effect of low-molecular-weight heparin.

REFERENCE

1) Broderick J, et al. Guidelines for the Management of Spontaneous Intracerebral Hemorrhage in Adults. *Stroke*. 2007;38:2001–2023.
2) Crowther MA, et al. Bleeding risk and the management of bleeding complications in patients undergoing anticoagulant therapy: focus on new anticoagulant agents. *BLOOD*. 2008;10:4871–4879.
3) Lexi-Comp, Inc. (Lexi-Drugs™). Lexi-Comp, Inc. 2010.

How do I treat beta-blocker overdose?

KEY CONCEPT	The treatment of beta-blocker overdose is focused at the reversal of symptoms and stabilization of heart rate and blood pressure.
HISTORY	**HPI:** Patient taking beta-blockers. Elderly patients with polypharmacy are at particular risk for accidental overdose. Sudden decompensation (syncope, dyspnea, hypoglycemia, delirium, coma). **PMH:** Hypertension, coronary artery disease, congestive heart failure, any indication for beta blockade.
PHYSICAL EXAM	Hypotension, bradycardia, seizure, delirium lethargy, unresponsive.
ELECTRO-CARDIOGRAM	Bradycardia, AV block, wide QRS, prolonged QTc, PR prolongation, asystole.
SYNTHESIS	**BB-OD** = Patient with suspected beta-blocker overdose. **BC** = Significant bradycardia: Ventricular rate < 55 bpm. May occur in setting of AV block. **HU** = **H**emodynamically **U**nstable: hypotension (systolic BP < 90 mm Hg) and evidence of shock (mental status changes or decreased urine output). **HS** = **H**emodynamically **S**table: normotensive, normal mentation, no evidence of shock. **STAB** = **STAB**ilize: For hypotension, start an IV fluid bolus with normal saline. Give glucagon 5 mg over 1 minute. If glucagon effective start glucagon infusion at 2–5 mg/hr to keep MAP >= 60. If necessary start inotropes with beta agonist activity to maintain blood pressure (epinephrine 1 mcg/min or dopamine 5 mcg/kg/min and titrate up to MAP >= 60). **INC-HR** = Increase heart rate: Give atropine 0.5–1mg every 5 minutes IV × 2 and assess response. Can use inotrope with beta agonist activity as above. Can use temporary pacing if above measures fail with either transcutaneous or transvenous pacing. **MED-TX** = Medical management: Monitor patients on telemetry. For hypoglycemia give an ampule of IV dextrose (D50W) and reassess. For seizures, break with IV or IM benzodiazepines (ex. lorazepam 2 mg IV). For patients with beta-blocker ingestion within 2 hours, give activated charcoal 1 g/kg by mouth if no contraindications. As the beta blocker drug levels wear off, decrease measures taken (ex. epinephrine infusion) as the clinical picture improves.
E **EPIPHANY**	**BB-OD + BC + HU = STAB + INC-HR + MED-TX** **BB-OD + BC + HS = MED-TX**

DISCUSSION	Beta-blocker toxicity occurs within 2 hours of ingestion in most patients. Treatment of beta-blocker toxicity should begin with evaluation of ABCs before proceeding with medical treatment. The goal of medical treatment is to reverse symptoms and stabilize blood pressure.
CONTRA-INDICATIONS	– Nausea and vomiting can occur as a side effect of glucagon. – Activated charcoal is contraindicated if patient is unable to protect the airway.
PEARLS	– Propranolol and carvedilol are highly lipophilic and can cross the blood-brain barrier to cause neurological sequelae such as seizures or delirium.
REFERENCE	1) Love JN, et al. Characterization of fatal beta blocker ingestion. *J Toxicol Clin Toxicol.* 2000;38(3):275–281. 2) Reith DM, et al. Relative toxicity of beta blockers in overdose. *J Toxicol Clin Toxicol.* 1996;34(3):273–278.

How do I manage digoxin toxicity?

 KEY CONCEPT	The management of an elevated digoxin level is based on the presence of symptoms and serum digoxin concentration.
 HISTORY	HPI: Patient taking digoxin for congestive heart failure (CHF) and/or atrial fibrillation (rate control). PMH: Renal insufficiency, hypothyroidism. Labs: Hypokalemia, hypomagnesemia, BUN, creatinine.
 PHYSICAL EXAM	Nausea, vomiting, diarrhea, visual disturbances (blurred or yellow vision), confusion, agitation.
 ELECTRO-CARDIOGRAM	Atrioventricular block, sinoatrial block, ventricular bigeminy, tachycardia, ventricular fibrillation.
 SYNTHESIS	**E-DIG** = **E**Levated serum **DIG**oxin > 2 ng/mL. **SYM** = **SYM**ptomatic: nausea, vomiting, visual disturbance (blurred or yellow vision), confusion, arrhythmia. **ASYM** = **ASYM**ptomatic: no symptoms present. **KN** = **KN**own level: known serum digoxin concentration. **UNKN** = **UNKN**own level: unknown serum digoxin concentration. **FAB** = Digoxin immune **FAB**. **HOLD** = Stop digoxin. **CAL-FAB** = **CAL**culated **FAB** dose [# vials] = (serum digoxin concentration [ng/mL] × weight [kg])/100 **10V** = **10 V**ials = 10 vials of Fab **HYPOK** = **HYPOK**alemia LOW K levels. **KREP** = Potassium (**K**) **REP**lacement: IV potassium at 10 to 20 mEq/hr (daily maximum 400 mEq/day) to maintain serum potassium levels between 4.0 and 5.5 mmol/L. **MGREP** = Ma**G**nesium **REP**lacement: give magnesium IV bolus 2 g over 15 minutes, followed by a continuous IV infusion (maximum 4 g/24 hours, including loading dose), as required. Maintain magnesium levels between 1.7 and 2.1 mg/dL.
E EPIPHANY	**Management of elevated digoxin:** **E-DIG + ASYM = HOLD** **SYM + KN = CAL-FAB** **SYM + UNKN = 10V** **Management of Electrolytes:** **HYPOK = KREP** **HYPOMG = MGREP**

DISCUSSION	Patients exhibiting symptoms of digoxin toxicity should be treated with Fab based on their serum digoxin concentrations. For severe, life-threatening toxicity, digoxin immune Fab is the treatment of choice. Low levels of potassium and magnesium should be corrected as these can exacerbate digoxin toxicity.
CONTRA-INDICATIONS	Drug-drug interactions that increase serum digoxin concentration: amiodarone, clarithromycin, cyclosporine, diltiazem, erythromycin, itraconazole, verapamil.
PEARLS	– Re-treatment with digoxin should not be resumed until all the Fab has been eliminated from the body. – Digoxin level may be falsely elevated after receiving Fab as the lab assay cannot distinguish between free digoxin and digoxin bound to Fab.
REFERENCE	1) Digoxin (Lanoxin) Package Insert— Glaxosmith Kline, September 2001. 2) Allen NM, et al. Treatment of digitalis intoxication with emphasis on the clinical use of digoxin immune Fab. *DICP* 1990;24(10):991–998. 3) Hauptman PJ, et al. Digitalis. *Circulation*. 1999;99;1265–1270.

Will this medication prolong the QT-c interval and how high is the risk?

KEY CONCEPT	Common medications can prolong the QT-c interval and lead to torsades de pointes (TDP), a life-threatening arrhythmia.
HISTORY	HPI: Patient with drug-induced prolongation of QT-c interval can exhibit palpitations, syncope, seizures, and/or cardiac arrest. PMH: Congenital long QT syndrome (LQTS), bradycardia, electrolyte imbalance (K, Mg), atrial fibrillation, congestive heart failure. SH: Age >65, female gender, alcohol. Meds: Digitalis, use of >2 QT prolonging drugs.
ELECTRO-CARDIOGRAM	Normal QT-c: 0.43 seconds in males and 0.45 seconds in females. Prolonged QT-c: 0.45 seconds in males and 0.47 seconds in females. TDP: Polymorphic Vtach, undulating rotations of QRS complex around ECG baseline.
SYNTHESIS	**QT-c** = Heart rate corrected QT interval, Bazzett formula for corrected QT = QT/[RR^0.5]. **HR** = **H**igh **R**isk: drugs that cause QT-c prolongation and have an increased of risk of TDP. **RA** = **R**isk **A**ssociation: drugs that cause QT-c prolongation and may be associated with TDP. **CR** = **C**ombination **R**isk: drugs that have a risk of QT-c prolongation and TDP under conditions such as (LQTS), overdose or in combination with other drugs causing prolonged QT-c.
E EPIPHANY	**Categories of QT-c prolonging drugs:** **HR: Amiodarone, clarithromycin, disopyramide, dofetilide, erythromycin, haloperidol, ibutilide, methadone, procainamide, quinidine, sotalol, thioridazine.** **RA: Amantadine, azithromycin, clozapine, dolasetron, flecainide, fosphenytoin, indapamide, isradipine, levofloxacin, lithium, moxifloxacin, nicardipine, ondansetron, perflutren, quetiapine, ranolazine, risperidone, vardenafil, venlafaxine, voriconazole.** **CR: Amitriptyline, ciprofloxacin, citalopram, fluconazole, fluoxetine, itraconazole, ketoconazole, mexilitine, nortriptyline, paroxetine, sertraline, trimethoprim-sulfamethoxazole**
DISCUSSION	A patient's risk for prolonged QT-c and TDP should be taken into consideration when initiating a drug with these potential side effects.

 PEARLS	– QT-c >0.5 seconds is high risk for ventricular arrhythmias/TDP. – With TDP check magnesium and potassium along with other causes.
REFERENCE	1) Arizona CERT. QT Drug Lists. www.qtdrugs.org 2) Roden DM. Drug-induced prolongation of the QT interval. *N Engl J Med.* 2004;350:1013–1022. 3) Goldenberg I, Arthur Moss. Long QT Syndrome *J Cardiovasc Electrophysiol.* 2006;17:333–336.

How do I manage a patient with heparin-induced thrombocytopenia?

KEY CONCEPT	Complication from heparin therapy causing a drop in platelet count and subsequently thrombosis by platelet activation.
HISTORY	Patient received UnFractionated Heparin (UFH) and has drop in platelet count 5–14 days after exposure. If rapid onset patients can appear septic within hours.
PHYSICAL EXAM	Fever/chills, hypertension, tachycardia, tachypnea, chest pain, skin rash, MI, stroke, peripheral ischemia, enlarging DVT, PE.
IMAGING	Doppler sonography to identify DVT.
SYNTHESIS	**DVT** = **D**eep **V**enous **T**hrombosis. **PE** = **P**ulmonary **E**mbolism. **DTI-3MO** = Begin **D**irect **T**hrombin **I**nhibitors and continue for **3 MO**nths; give agatroban if renal dysfunction, lepirudin if liver dysfunction, either if no renal/liver dysfunction. **DTI-6MO** = Begin **D**irect **T**hrombin **I**nhibitors and continue for **6 MO**nths; give agatroban if renal dysfunction, lepirudin if liver dysfunction, either if no renal/liver dysfunction. **HIT-POS** = **HIT POS**itive serology. **HIT-NEG** = **HIT NEG**ative serology **LMWH** = **L**ow **M**olecular **W**eight (lovenox). **UFH** = Unfractionated heparin. **STOP-HEP** = **STOP HEP**arin (either LMWH or UFH). **HEP** = Give or continue with **HEP**arin (either LMWH or UFH). **TCP** = **T**hrombo**C**yto**P**enia (reduction in platelets of >= 50% from baseline). **LOOK** = **LOOK** for and work-up for an alternative cause of TCP, eg, sepsis. **WAR** = **WAR**farin. **STOP-UN-WAR** = **STOP UN**opposed **W**arfarin (ie, warfarin being given without any other anticoagulant such as HEP or DTI. **PLT-TRANS** = Begin **PL**a**T**elet **TRANS**fusion. **BLEED** = Patient is actively **BLEED**ing.
E **EPIPHANY**	**HIT-POS = STOP-HEP + STOP-UN-WAR + DTI-3MO** **HIT-NEG = HEP** **HIT-NEG + TCP = LOOK** **HIT-POS + TCP + BLEED = PLT-TRANS** **HIT-POS + DVT/PE = DTI-6MO**

DISCUSSION	Type II (immune-mediated) HIT = the clinically important HIT, which causes a moderate to severe reduction in platelet count, is antibody-mediated, and clinically results in a high risk for thrombosis. Diagnose with platelet count and ELISA antibodies against heparin PF4 complexes and serotonin release assay. HIT antibodies disappear in 3 months of stopping heparin; once antibodies are cleared the risk for HIT is no higher than patients with no history of HIT. In patients with HIT undergoing PIC for ACS, argatroban with or without GPIIb/IIIa provides adequate anticoagulation and is well tolerated.
PEARLS	– HIT typically occurs 5–10 days after heparin administration. – DTI: lepirudin cleared renal, argatroban cleared hepatically, monitor PTT. – Stratify based on T score: thrombocytopenia, timing, thrombosis, alternative causes.
REFERENCE	1) Douketis JD. Perioperative anticoagulation management in patients hwo are receiving oral anticoagulant therapy: a practical guide for clinicians. *Throm Res.* 2002;108:3. 2) Warkentin TE. Heparin-induced thrombocytopenia: pathogenesis and management. *Br J Haematol.* 2003;121:535.

What are the side effects and complications of certain cardiovascular medications?

KEY CONCEPT	Medication side effect and adverse reactions are a major cause of hospital admission and death.
HISTORY	A patient that presents with a medication reaction that is harmful and unintended at doses normally used for therapy.
PHYSICAL EXAM	Mental status, uremia, encephalopathy, hepatomegaly, cirrhosis, liver failure, jaundice, icterus, thyromegaly, age, body habitus.
ELECTRO-CARDIOGRAM	Heart rate, PR, OTc, QRS interval prolongation, peaked T waves, ST changes.
SYNTHESIS (cont. on next page)	**HEP** = **HEP**arin and fibrinolytics. **B-HIT** = **B**leeding, monitor PTT, **H**eparin-**I**nduced **T**hrombocytopenia. **ASA/PLAV** = **A**spirin, **PLAV**ix, glycoprotein IIb/IIIA, and anticoagulants. **TIC** = **TIC**lopidine. **AA-TTP-N** = **A**plastic **A**nemia, **TTP**, **N**eutropenia. **AC-NI** = **A**nti**C**holingeric side effects, **N**egative **I**notrope. **SN-CYP** = **S**kin **N**ecrosis, wide range of **CYP** interactions (inhibit and induce). **INC-DIG** = **INC**reases **DIG**oxin levels. **LLS** = **L**upus-**L**ike **S**yndrome. **B-H-V-T-L-P** = **B**radycardia, **H**ypotension, **V**isual changes, **T**hyroid disease, **L**iver toxicity, and **P**ulmonary fibrosis. **DNU-K-C-T-M** = **D**o **N**ot **U**se with **K**etoconazole, **C**imetidine, **T**rimethorpim, **M**egestrol. **HVO-E-HU** = **H**ypo**V**olemia, **E**lectrolyte disturbances, **H**yper**U**ricemia. **HYPERK** = **HYPERK**alemia. **STRUC** = Not be used with known **STRUC**tural heart disease. **PE** = **P**eripheral **E**dema. **HTox-MTox** = **H**epato**T**oxicity, **M**yo**T**oxicity, avoid with grapefruit juice. **EOS-HTN** = **EOS**inophilia, **H**yper**T**ensio**N** with beta blockers. **C-LI-HK-ARF** = **C**ough, increased **LI**thium levels, **H**yper**K**alemia, **A**cute **R**enal **F**ailure. **BC-AVB** = **B**rady**C**ardia/first degree **AV B**lock. **PH** = **P**ostural **H**ypotension. **COU** = **COU**madin. **QUIN** = **QUIN**idine.

SYNTHESIS (cont. from previous page)	**PROC** = **PROC**ainamide. **DISO** = **DISO**pyramide. **FLEC** = **FLEC**anide. **AMIO** = **AMIO**darone. **DOFET** = **DOFET**ilide. **TDZ** = **T**hiazide. **LOOP** = **LOOP** diurectics. **K** = **P**otassium sparing. **BB** = **B**eta **B**lockers. **AB** = **A**lpha **B**lockers: **CCB** = **C**alcium **B**lockers (diltiazem/verapamil). **DHP** = **D**i**H**ydro**P**yridines. **ACEI** = **ACE I**nhibitors. **VAS** = **VAS**odilators (hydralazine, minoxidil). **STAT** = **STAT**ins. **DOB** = **DOB**utamine.
E EPIPHANY	**HEP: B-HIT** **ASA/PLAV: B** **TIC: AA-TTP-N** **COU: SN-CYP** **QUIN: INC-DIG** **PROC: LLS** **DISO: AC-NI** **FLEC: STRUC** **AMIO: B-H-V-T-L-P** **DOFET: DNU-K-C-T-M** **TDZ: HVO-E-HU** **LOOP: HVO** **K: HYPERK** **BB: BC-AVB** **AB: PH** **CCB: DIG** **DHP: PE** **ACEI: C-LI-HK-ARF** **VAS: PE** **STAT: HTox-MTox** **DOB: EOS-HTN**
DISCUSSION	Patients with heart disease are at risk for adverse drug reactions because the disease process can influence drug metabolism and elimination via changes in liver and kidney perfusion. These patients are also likely to have advance age–associated changes in metabolism and polypharmacy.
REFERENCE	1) Opie LH, Gersh BJ. *Drugs for the Heart*. 6th ed. Philadelphia, PA: Saunder's; 2005. 2) O'Rourke R, Walsh R, Fuster V. *Hursts's The Heart, Manual of Cardiology*. 12th ed. New York: McGraw-Hill; 2008.

Which inotropes and vasopressors do I use for my patient in shock?

KEY CONCEPT	Vasopressors and inotropes (positive/negative) are used for management of cardiovascular conditions—shock/heart failure. The choice of agent depends on specific pharmacological effects and the condition of the patient.
HISTORY	Fatigue, altered mental status, weakness, diaphoresis, chest pain, diarrhea.
PHYSICAL EXAM	CV: Tachycardia, narrow pulse pressure, hypotension, weak pulses. Resp: Rapid shallow respiration. Renal: Low urine output. Ext: Cold clammy skin
IMAGING	Refer to Swan–Ganz chapter for interpretations of readings.
SYNTHESIS	**CG-SHOCK** = **C**ardio**G**enic **SHOCK**. **SEP-SHOCK** = **SEP**tic **SHOCK**. **VAS** = **VAS**opressors (dopamine, epinephrine, norepinephrine, phenylephrine, vasopressin). **INO** = **INO**tropes (dobutamine, milrinone). **DA** = **D**op**A**mine start at 2.5 mcg/kg/min; titrate dose over range of 0.5–20 mcg/kg/min for effect. **NE** = **N**orepin**E**phrine start at 0.1 mcg/kg/min; titrate dose over range of 0.1–1 mcg/kg/min for effect. **PE** = **P**henyl**E**phrine start at 01.0 mcg/kg/min; titrate dose over range of 0.5–5 mcg/kg/min for effect. **EP** = **E**pinephrine start at 0.05 mcg/kg/min; titrate dose over range of 0.03–0.1 mcg/kg/min for effect. **VP** = **V**aso**P**ressin start at 0.04 units/min; titrate dose over range of 0.01–0.07 units/min for effect. **DB** = **D**o**B**utamine start at 5 mcg/kg/min; titrate dose over range of 2.5–20 mcg/kg/min for effect. **MR** = **M**il**R**inone start at 0.50 mcg/kg/min; titrate dose over range of 0.375–0.75 mcg/kg/min for effect.
EPIPHANY	**CG-SHOCK = INO or DA/EP** **SEP-SHOCK = VAS**
DISCUSSION	The types of shock dictate the treatment and include hypovolemic, cardiogenic, distributive (septic, anaphylactic, neurogenic).

PEARLS	The severity of shock is based on the loss of blood volume and is graded from stage 1–4: Stage 1: 15% (750 mL) Stage 2: 15–30% (750–1500 mL) Stage 3: 30–40% (1500–2000 mL) Stage 4: 40–50% (>2 liters)
REFERENCE	1) Mullner M, Urbanek B, Havel C, et al. Vasopressors for shock. *Cochrane Database Syst Rev.* 2004 Nov;32(11 Suppl):S455–465. 2) Lollgen H, Drexler H. Use of inotropes in the critical care setting. *Crit Care Med.* 1990 Jan;18(1 Pt 2):S56–S60.

Which IV antihypertensive do I use?

KEY CONCEPT	There are many classes of IV antihypertensives that lower blood pressure via different mechanisms; the ultimate goal is to prevent the endpoint of end organ damage.
HISTORY	Patient unable to take or tolerate oral therapy who presents with cerebral infarction, pulmonary edema, hypertensive emergency, encephalopathy, CHF, ICH, aortic dissection, eclampsia.
PHYSICAL EXAM	Neuro: Altered mental status, encephalopathy, fatigue, seizures. CV: Chest pain. RESP: SOB, tachypnea.
IMAGING	Refer to the additional table for hemodynamic effects in the Swan–Ganz chapter.
SYNTHESIS	**HF** = **H**eart **F**ailure. **HTN** = **H**yper**T**ensio**N**. **HTN-EM** = **H**yper**T**ensio**N** **EM**ergency. **ISCH** = **ISCH**emia. **PREG** = **PREG**nancy/Eclampsia. **VEN** = **VEN**ous vasodilators. Sodium Nitroprusside: start at 0.25 mcg/kg/min, and titrate every 5 minutes up to a maximum of 10 mcg/kg/min. Or Nitroglcerin: initially 2.5 mcg/kg/min, and titrate every 5 minutes up to a maximum of 200 mcg/min. **BETA** = **BETA** blockers. Labetalol 20 mg IV bolus, then repeat and uptitrate dose every 10 minutes (maxium 8 0 mg) until effect, then repeat every 6 hours (alternatively, following bolus, begin drip at 0.5 mg/min and titrate for effect up to a maximum of 2 mg/min). Or Esmolol 500 mcg/kg bolus, then start infusion at 50 mcg/g/min, uptitrate every 5 minutes for effect up to a maximum of 300 mcg/kg/min. **CCB** = **C**alcium **C**hannel **B**lockers. Nicardipine begin at 5 mg/hr, and uptitrate by 2.5 mg/hr every 5 minutes for effect up to a maximum dose of 15 mg/hr. Or Diltiazem initial 15 mg bolus, then begin infusion at 5 mg/hr, and uptitrate every 5 minutes for effect up to a maximum of 15 mg/hr. Or Verapamil 5 mg IV bolus, then uptitrate every 4 hours in increments of 2.5 mg for effect, up to a maximum of 10 mg IV every 6 hours. **A-VAS** = **A**rterial/**VAS**odilators. Hydralazine 10 mg IV/IM bolus, then uptitrate in 10 mg increments every 6 hours for effect, with a maximum dose of 50 mg IV/IM every 6 hours.

 EPIPHANY	**HTN + HF/ISCH = VEN/BETA** **HTN-EM = BETA/CCB** **HTN + PREG = A-VAS**
 DISCUSSION	The agent of choice should be based on the desired hemodynamic effect, side effect, and availability.
 PEARLS	– Oral agents lower blood pressure slower than parenteral forms.
 REFERENCE	1) Zigmont EA, Connelly JF. Intravenous antihypertensive agents for patients unable to take oral medications. *Am J Health Syst Pharm*. 1995 Jul 15;52(14):1514–1516.

How do I convert these cardiac medications from IV to PO?

⌐O KEY CONCEPT	HPI: Can the patient swallow pills or does he/she have a feeding tube?
🩺 PHYSICAL EXAM	Vitals: Are the BP and HR under control at the current dose(s)?
⧖ SYNTHESIS	**ENAL** = **ENAL**april. **FUR** = **FUR**osemide. **HYD** = **HYD**ralazine. **LABE** = **LABE**talol. **LEVTHY** = **LEVOTHY**roxine. **MET** = **MET**oprolol tartrate.
E EPIPHANY	**IV to PO RATIO: #:#** **ENAL = 1:8** **FUR = 1:2** **HYD = 1:2** **LABE = 1:4** **LEVTHY = 1:2** **MET = 1:2.5**

PEARLS	– Pills which that should not be crushed include the following: – Nifedipine extended- release (Procardia XL®), use amlodipine (Norvasc®) instead. – Immediate-release nifedipine is NOT recommended due to the potential for sudden decrease in blood pressure that may cause coronary steal or stroke. – Isosorbide mononitrate (Imdur®), use isosoribide dinitrate (Isordil®) instead. – Metoprolol succinate (Toprol XL®), use metoprolol tartrate (Lopressor®) instead. – Metoprolol succinate may be cut in half, but may not be crushed.
REFERENCE	1) Lexi-Comp, Inc. (Lexi-Drugs™). Lexi-Comp, Inc. May 1, 2009.

Which cardiac medications can be used during pregnancy and lactation?

KEY CONCEPT	The FDA has an assessment of the risk of fetal injury due to the pharmaceutical if taken by the mother during pregnancy.
HISTORY	HPI: How many weeks of gestation is the patient?
SYNTHESIS	**A: Pregnancy Category A = SAFE** = Human studies show no risk to fetus in 1st trimester and there is no evidence of risk in later trimesters. **B: Pregnancy Category B = PROBABLY SAFE** = Animal reproduction studies have failed to demonstrate a risk to the fetus, and there are no adequate and well-controlled studies in pregnant women OR Animal studies have shown an adverse effect, but adequate and well-controlled studies in pregnant women have failed to demonstrate a risk to the fetus in any trimester **C: Pregnancy Category C = PROBABLY A RISK BUT BENEFITS MAY OUTWEIGH** = Animal reproduction studies have shown an adverse effect on the fetus and there are no adequate and well-controlled studies in humans, but potential benefits may warrant use of the drug in pregnant women despite potential risks. **D: Pregnancy Category D = RISK OCCURS BUT HIGH BENEFITS MAY OUTWEIGH RISK** = There is positive evidence of human fetal risk based on adverse reaction data from investigational or marketing experience or studies in humans, but potential benefits may warrant use of the drug in pregnant women despite potential risks. **X: Pregnancy Category X = SEVERE RISK = DON'T USE EVER.** **BFY:** Breast Feeding Ok, **BFN:** Breast Feeding Not OK, **BFU:** Unknown. **AMIO:** Amiodarone, **AML:** Amlodipine, **ASA:** Aspirin, **ATEN:** Atenolol. **ATOR:** Atorvastatin, **CAPT:** Captopril, **CARV:** Carvedilol, **DIG:** Digoxin. **DILT:** Diltiazem, **ENAL:** Enalapril, **FLEC:** Flecanide, **FUR:** Furosemide. **HYDR:** Hydralazine, **LABE:** Labetalol, **LIDO:** Lidocaine, **LISIN:** Lisinopril. **MDOPA:** Methyldopa, **METO:** Metoprolol, **NIFED:** Nifedipine, **PROC:** Procainamide, **PROPF:** Propafenone, **PROP:** Propranolol, **Q:** Quinidine. **SIM:** Simvastatin, **SOT:** Sotalol, **VERA:** Verapamil, **WAR:** Warfarin.
E EPIPHANY (cont. on next page)	**AMIO = D + BFN** **AML = C + BFU** **ASA = C + BFY (low doses)** **ATEN = D + BFY (caution—bradycardia)** **ATOR = X + BFN** **CAPT = C/D 2–3rd trimester + BFY** **CARV = C/D 2–3rd trimester + BFU** **DIG = C + BFY** **DILT = C + BFU** **ENAL = C/D 2–3rd trimester + BFY**

E EPIPHANY (cont. from previous page)	FLEC = C + BFY FUR = C + BFY HYDR = C + BFY LABE = C + BFY LIDO = B + BFY LISIN = C/D 2–3rd trimester + BFY DOPA = B + BFY METO = C/D 2–3rd trimester + BFY NIFED = C + BFU PROC = C + BFY PROPF = C + BFU PROP = C/D 2–3rd trimester + BFU Q = C + BFY SIM = X + BFN SOT = B/D 2–3rd trimester + BFU VERA = C + BFY WAR = D/X + BFY
DISCUSSION	Prenatal vitamins are safe to take during pregnancy; herbal medications have NOT been proven safe.
PEARLS	– Pregnancy Category X: Studies in animals or humans have demonstrated fetal abnormalities, and/or there is positive evidence of human fetal risk based on adverse reaction data from investigational or marketing experience, and the risks involved in use of the drug in pregnant women clearly outweigh potential benefits.
REFERENCE	1) Sannerstedt R, Lundborg P, Danielsson BR, et al. (February 1996). "Drugs during pregnancy: an issue of risk classification and information to prescribers". *Drug Saf.* 14(2):69–77. 2) Zipes D, Braunwald E. *Braunwald's Heart Disease.* 8th ed. Chicago: Saunders. 3) Briggs G, Freeman R, Yaffe S. *Drugs in Pregnancy and Lactation.* 7th ed. Philadelphia: Lippincott Williams Wilkins.

242 MEDICATIONS

What should I do for patients scheduled to receive contrast who have a contrast or dye allergy?

KEY CONCEPT

Hypersensitivity reactions occur most frequently with high-osmolar, ionic contrast media and least frequently with low-osmolar, nonionic contrast media. Pruritus and urticaria are the most common hypersensitivity reactions.

HISTORY

HPI: What type of reaction did the patient have?
What type of contrast agent was given?
How long ago was the reaction?

PHYSICAL EXAM

Altered mental status.
Pruritis, urticaria.
Tachycardia.
Tachypnea.
Nausea/vomiting/diarrhea.

SYNTHESIS

ELCE = **EL**ective **C**ontrast **E**xposure.
URCE = **UR**gent **C**ontrast **E**xposure.
IVNS-EL = **IV N**ormal **S**aline (0.9% saline) at 1 mg/kg/hr for at least 2 hours before and 12 hours after contrast exposure in patients with no current signs/symptoms of heart failure or volume overload.
PRED-EL = Give prednisone 50 mg orally 12 hours and 2 hours prior to contrast exposure.
DPHD-EL = **D**i**P**hen**H**y**D**ramine 50 mg orally 12 hours and 2 hours prior to contrast exposure.
FAMO-EL = **FAMO**tidine 20 mg orally 12 hours and 2 hours prior to contrast exposure.
DMMP-UR = **D**exa**M**ethasone 8 mg IV or **M**ethyl**P**rednisonlone 40 mg IV given **UR**gently immediately prior to contrast exposure.
DPHD-UR = **D**i**P**hen**H**y**D**ramine 50 mg IV given **UR**gently immediately prior to contrast exposure.
FAMO-UR = **FAMO**tidine 20 mg IV given **UR**gently immediately prior to contrast exposure.

E

EPIPHANY

ELCE = IVNS-EL + PRED-EL + DPHD-EL + FAMO-EL
URCE = DMMP-UR + DPHD-UR + FAMO-UR

DISCUSSION	Sixty percent of patients with a previous hypersensitivity reaction to contrast media have repeat reaction when reexposed. The contrast exposure should preferably use low-osmolar contrast media if possible to minimize risk of re-reaction. The death rate related to contrast allergy is rare (about 1 in 40,000 cases).
REFERENCE	1) Brockow K, Christiansen C, Kanny G, Clement O, Barbaud A, et al. Management of hypersensitivity reactions to iodinated contrast media. *Allergy*. 2005;60:150–158.

If there is an interacting medication, what dose should I start amiodarone at in this patient?

KEY CONCEPT	Amiodarone is a class III antiarrhythmic medication which can interact with other drugs and increase the probability of adverse effects.
HISTORY	HPI: Patient taking amiodarone or starting amiodarone. PMH: Heart failure, pulmonary disease, liver disease, thyroid disease. SH: Alcohol, smoking.
PHYSICAL EXAM	Palpitations, chest pain, dyspnea fatigue.
ELECTRO-CARDIOGRAM	Prolonged QT interval.
SYNTHESIS	**AMIO** = **AMIO**darone **QTD** = **QT D**rugs: These are drugs known to prolong the QT interval and the effect is potentiated with the addition of amiodarone. A prolonged QT interval increases the probability of Torsades de Pointes, which can be lethal. See QTc chapter for list of QT prolonging drugs. Classic examples include azole antifungals, fluoroquinolones, macrolides, quinidine, and procainamide. **AVN** = **AV N**odal agents: These are drugs that have a negative chronotropic effect and/or slow conduction through the AV node. This effect is potentiated by the addition of amiodarone and can result in severe bradycardia or high degree AV block. Classic drugs in this class are beta blockers and calcium channel blockers such as diltiazem. **CSA** = Cyclosporine: with AMIO elevates cyclosporine and creatinine levels. **DIG** = **DIG**oxin: with AMIO elevates digoxin levels. **PNY** = **PH**en**Y**toin: with AMIO increases phenytoin levels. **WAR** = **WAR**farin = with AMIO increases INR. **AVOID** = **AVOID** combination if possible. If it is not possible to avoid the combination use MONITOR as a less optimal approach. **HALF** = **HALF** dose: Decrease AMIO dose by 50%. **MONITOR** = **MONITOR** the effect of AMIO, particularly heart rate, QTc interval, and PR interval. For medications such as CSA, DIG, PNY, and WAR, check the resulting drug level/INR. Decrease AMIO dose and/or the dose of the interacting medication as necessary.
EPIPHANY	**AMIO + QTD = AVOID** **AMIO + AVN = MONITOR** **AMIO + DIG / WAR = HALF + MONITOR** **AMIO + CSA / PNY = HALF + MONITOR**

DISCUSSION	Amiodarone is an inhibitor of the cytochrome P450 3A4 enzyme system and p-glycoprotein, leading to numerous drug–drug interactions. It is broken down and excreted solely by the liver with a half life of 60 days.
CONTRA-INDICATIONS	**Do not begin AMIO if:** – Cardiogenic shock. – Marked sinus bradycardia. – Second or third degree atrioventricular block. – Known hypersensitivity to amiodarone or iodine.
PEARLS	– There are numerous serious adverse effects associated with amiodarone therapy, including: AV block, bradycardia, congestive heart failure, hypersensitivity pneumonitis, pulmonary fibrosis, hyperthyroidism, hypothyroidism, liver failure, optic neuritis, visual disturbances.
REFERENCE	1) Amiodarone (Cordarone) Package Insert – Wyeth Pharmaceuticals, May 2009. 2) Chitwood KK, et al. Cyclosporin-amiodarone interaction. *Ann Pharmacother.* 1993;27(5):569–571. 3) Arizona CERT. QT Drug Lists. www.qtdrugs.org.

Which diuretic should I use if my patient has a sulfa allergy?

KEY CONCEPT	Anaphylaxis may develop with repeat exposure to allergens such as sulfa.
HISTORY	HPI: Description of allergic reaction, temporal relationship between reaction and medications, concomitant allergies. Allergic reaction presents most commonly as either a maculopapular eruption or an urticarial rash that develops within 1–3 days of initial medication administration and resolves spontaneously upon discontinuation of the drug. Anaphylaxis may develop with repeat exposure. There is a dreaded delayed hypersensitivity response (Stevens Johnson syndrome) that can occur as a consequence of sulfa drugs. The incidence is rare and unfortunately there is no good way to predict who will succumb.
SYNTHESIS	**MILD SULFA** = patient with **MILD SULFA** allergy. Mild pruritis or urticaria with another sulfa-containing medication would fall into this group. **SEV SULFA** = patient with **SEV**ere **SULFA** allergy. Any patient who had anaphylaxis or something similar to Stevens-Johnson syndrome automatically falls into this group and should not be given sulfa. **LD** = **L**oop **D**iuretics with sulfa (ex. furosemide, torsemide, bumetanide) **TD** = **T**hiazide **D**iuretics are unlikely to trigger an allergic reaction in patients with sulfa allergy and can be used safely in those patients (ex. hydrochlorothiazide, chlorothiazide, metolazone) **EA** = **E**thacrynic **A**cid = the only loop diuretic which does not contain a sulfonamide molecule and may be considered in patients with severe sulfa allergy.
EPIPHANY	**MILD SULFA = LD or TD** **SEV SULFA = EA or TD**
DISCUSSION	Loop Diuretics have a low cross-reactivity to the sulfa moiety in other medications such as antibiotics that more commonly cause allergy and can be tried in patients with mild allergy. Ethacrynic acid is the only loop diuretic that does not contain a sulfonamide molecule and may be considered in those patients with severe allergic reactions. Sulfa allergies are commonly linked to medications that contain a sulfonamide molecule. However, there are distinct groups of sulfonamides: (1) Sulfonylarylamines—Includes sulfa antibiotics (trimethoprim-sulfamethoxazole, sulfisoxazole, Dapsone). (2) Non-sulfonylarylamines—Includes carbonic anhydrase inhibitors (acetazolamide), loop diuretics (furosemide, bumetanide, torsemide), thiazide diuretics (hydrochlorothiazide), sulfonylureas (glyburide, glipizide), COX-2 inhibitors, protease inhibitors. (3) Sulfonamide moiety-containing—Includes ibutalide, sotalol, sumatript.

PEARLS	– Patients with serious allergic reactions to medications and/or multiple drug allergies may be at an increased risk for hypersensitivity reactions despite the low risk of cross-reactivity.
REFERENCE	1) Johnson JJ, Green DL, Rife JP, Limon L. Sulfonamide cross-reactivity: fact or fiction? *Ann Pharmacother.* 2005;39:290–301. 2) Furosemide (Lasix®) Package Insert — Sanofi Aventis, September 2008. 3) Bumetanide Package Insert — Bedford Labs, June 2005.

INDEX

Page numbers followed by *f* or *t* indicate figures or tables, respectively.